Guide for the Development and Management of Nursing Libraries and Information Resources

Dorothy L. Moore, MS, RN

NLN Press • New York
Pub. No. 14-7297

Copyright © 1997
National League for Nursing Press
350 Hudson Street, New York, NY 10014

Library of Congress Cataloging-in-Publication Data

Moore, Dorothy L.
    Guide for the development and management of nursing libraries and information resources / Dorothy L. Moore.
        p.   cm.
    "Pub. no. 14-7297"
    Includes bibliographical references and index.
    ISBN 0-88737-729-7
    1. Nursing libraries—United States. I. Title.
    [DNLM: 1. Libraries, Nursing—organization & administration.
    2. Information Services—organization & administration. Z 675.N8
    M821g 1997]
    Z675.N8M66   1997
    025.1'9661073—dc21
    DNLM/DLC
    for Library of Congress   97-14566
                                                                           CIP

This book was set in Galliard and Garamond by Publications Development Company, Crockett, Texas. The editor and designer was Allan Graubard. BookCrafters was the printer.

Printed in the United States of America

Contents

Contributors

Richard Barry, MLS
Librarian
American Nurses Association
600 Maryland Ave., SW
Suite 100 West
Washington, DC 20024-2571
202-651-7413
E-mail: rbarry@ana.org

Dawn Bick, BNSc, MLS, AHIP
Assistant Executive Director
Houston Academy of Medicine—
    Texas Medical Center Library
1133 M.D. Anderson Blvd.
Houston, TX 77030-2809
713-799-7126
E-mail: dbick@library.tmc.edu

Jonathan DeForest Eldredge, MLS,
    PhD
Assistant Professor and Chief of
    Collections and Information
    Resources Development
Health Sciences Center Library
University of New Mexico
Albuquerque, NM 87131-5686
505-272-0654
E-mail: jeldredg@biblio.unm.edu

Deborah L. Graham, MLS
Assistant Director for Biomedical
    Information Services
Health Sciences Center Library
University of New Mexico
Albuquerque, NM 87131-5686
505-272-0639
E-mail: dgraham@biblio.unm.edu

Warren G. Hawkes, MLS, AHIP
Director, Library and Records
    Management
New York State Nurses Association
46 Cornell Road
Latham, NY 12110-1403
518-782-9400, ext. 227
E-mail: warren.hawkes@nysna.org

Margaret M. Jarrette, MLS
Catalog Librarian
Bibliographic Services
Samuel Paley Library
Temple University
Philadelphia, PA 19122

Craig Locatis, PhD
Education Research Specialist
Learning Center for Interactive
    Technology
National Library of Medicine
8600 Rockville Pike
Bethesda, MD 20894
301-435-3254
E-mail: locatis@nlm.nih.gov

Caroline E. Mann, MSLS
Portland Campus Librarian
Linfield College—Portland Campus
2255 NW Northrup
Portland, OR 97210
503-413-7820
E-mail: cmann@linfield.edu

Contributors

Dorothy L. Moore, MS, RN
Technical Information Specialist
National Library of Medicine
8600 Rockville Pike
Bethesda, MD 20894
301-496-6531
E-mail: dorothy__moore@ccmail
    .nlm.nih.gov

Julie M. Pavri, MSN, MLS
Associate Director
Library and Records Management
New York State Nurses Association
46 Cornell Road
Latham, NY 12110-1403
518-782-9400, ext. 229
E-mail: julie.pavri@nysna.org

Jacqueline Picciano, MSLS, MBA,
    FMLA, AHIP
Team Librarian
Information Services
Cornell Medical Library
1300 York Avenue
New York, NY 10021
212-746-6053
E-mail: jlpicci@med.cornell.edu

Diane Pravikoff, RN, MSN
Director of Research/Professional
    Liaison
Cinahl Information Systems
1509 Wilson Terrace, P.O. Box 871
Glendale, CA 91209-0871
818-409-8206
E-mail: dpravikoff@cinahl.com

Juliette Ratner, MS
Librarian
Mountainside Hospital
School of Nursing
Louise A. Mershon Library
Bay & Highland Avenues
Montclair, NJ 07042
201-429-6063

Karen Sinkule, AMLS
Preservation Information Librarian
Preservation and Collection
    Management Section
National Library of Medicine
8600 Rockville Pike
Bethesda, MD 20894
301-496-8124
E-mail: karen
    sinkule@ccmail.nlm.nih.gov

Debra L. Spunt, MS, RN
Manager, Clinical Simulation
    Laboratories
University of Maryland
School of Nursing
655 West Lombard Street
Baltimore, MD 21201
410-706-7898

Madeline Turkeltaub, RN, PhD,
    CRNP
Assistant Professor
University of Maryland
School of Nursing
655 West Lombard Street
Baltimore, MD 21201
410-706-4144

Michael Weisberg, EdD
Program Manager
Learning Center for Interactive
    Technology
National Library of Medicine
8600 Rockville Pike
Bethesda, MD 20894
301-435-3259
E-mail: weisberg@nlm.nih.gov

Sharon R. Willis, MLS
Cataloger
Cataloging Section
National Library of Medicine
8600 Rockville Pike
Bethesda, MD 20894
301-496-7138
E-mail: sharon
    willis@ccmail.nlm.nih.gov

Preface

This book is the culmination of a collaborative project undertaken by the Interagency Council on Information Resources for Nursing (ICIRN) and the National League for Nursing. The ICIRN is a voluntary group established in 1960 consisting of agencies and organizations interested in improving information services for nurses.

The purpose of this book is to provide information and guidance on developing and managing information resources and services for nurses in a variety of settings, including clinical units and centers, laboratories and learning resource centers, and nursing libraries in hospitals, colleges, and universities. It includes information that should be especially useful to deans, directors, and administrators of nursing programs, affiliated and unaffiliated nurses, as well as librarians and information specialists. This book is not a handbook, but the range of information included is broad in scope yet deals with those areas of primary concern in developing and managing nursing information resources. This book intends the following:

- To provide answers to frequent and recurring queries from nurses and nursing school librarians received by many of the chapter contributors and ICIRN representatives regarding information resources and services;

- To provide an overview of issues and practical advice relating to the development, management and provision of information services for nurses; and

- To enable persons responsible for nursing information resources to make a good start on locating sources of nursing information, or on developing, managing, evaluating, or extending resources and services.

Suggested readings on selected topics that were either discussed or mentioned in the chapters are included at the end of the chapters. These suggested readings either complement or supplement chapter information. The resource references, address lists, and other material at the end of the chapters are intended to assist users of this book in locating additional and more specific information for providing, developing, or managing resources. An effort has been made to include the most current information available at the time of the preparation of the manuscripts for the chapters in this book. However, as new revisions of listed publications and information appear, some of the resource references included and the Internet addresses should be adequate to enable users of this book to locate this information.

Each chapter covers discrete topics but is linked to other chapters in the book because of interrelated concepts and activities involved in providing information services. Chapter 1 provides a review of the trends in nursing education, clinical practice, and information needs of students and nurses in light of the changing health care delivery system and information technology; Chapters 2 and 3 address administrative issues in relation to the parent or sponsoring organization, such as services, budgeting, accreditation, and personnel management; Chapter 4 focuses on the provision of information and educational services; Chapter 5 provides virtually everything one needs to know on developing and evaluating nursing collections; Chapter 6 provides an overview of cataloging and processing materials with specific information relating to nursing materials; Chapter 7 gives valuable information on what to do about archival materials and where they may possibly be deposited; Chapter 8 provides information on preserving the library collection and where to get free advice; Chapter 9 covers audiovisuals, computer laboratories, and clinical simulation facilities; and Chapter 10 gives an overview of the programs and services of the National Library of Medicine that are available to health professionals and persons managing libraries in the health sciences.

ACKNOWLEDGMENTS

Special thanks to the chapter contributors for their generous efforts and commitment in sharing their experiences and knowledge on developing and managing information resources for nurses. The ICIRN is especially grateful to Warren Hawkes, Dawn Bick, and Richard Barry for reviewing many of the manuscripts that were submitted for this book. And finally, thanks to the National League for Nursing Press for making this publication possible and for its patience with the representatives and members of the member agencies of the ICIRN as they prepared the manuscript.

1

Introduction: Information Resources and Services for Nursing

Diane S. Pravikoff, RN, MSN
Warren G. Hawkes, MLS, AHIP

The information age, though still in its infancy, already has profoundly affected the manner in which institutions and individuals interact; the rudimentary nature of interpersonal relations and communications has changed forever (Axley, 1996). Concomitant with these societal changes is the rapid evolution of health care. Professionals within the health care delivery system are finding it difficult to establish educational paths and develop practice parameters to meet the demands of a constantly evolving system. This is particularly true for nurses, the single largest group of health care providers. The rapid shift away from the acute care setting, down-substitution of nurses with unlicensed assistive personnel, and an ever-increasing emphasis on the bottom line are issues of great concern within the nursing profession—to the extent that some question the viability of nursing itself (Monsen, 1996). To deter that process, nurses must be empowered as effective practitioners in any style of system that develops. Information and knowledge are the keys to that empowerment.

Diane S. Pravikoff & Warren G. Hawkes

It is essential that practitioners develop a basic understanding of the information resources related to their profession. In many cases, such as freestanding clinics and visiting nurse associations, practitioners will not have ready physical access to the type of resources they may have utilized during their educational program. Consequently, individual nurses will find it beneficial, even necessary, to develop a rudimentary understanding of the processes involved in accessing and using information resources. This chapter provides a framework for understanding the scope and level of information resources and services needed by nursing students in various educational programs and by licensed nurses in a variety of practice environments. Later chapters focus on more formal library structures, but the underlying principles of information acquisition, organization, and dissemination are equally applicable to a less formally structured information environment.

NURSING EDUCATION AND PRACTICE

Types of Educational Programs

Modern nursing education, founded on the principles of Florence Nightingale in the mid-nineteenth century, continues to undergo change. Initially, most education was conducted through apprenticeship arrangements in hospitals, but as progress was made in the science of medicine, with resultant changes in the delivery of care, it became obvious that nurses needed more formalized training and education (Rush, 1992). Schools of nursing, generally affiliated with hospitals, were established, with student nurses functioning as hospital staff as part of their education.

University education for nurses began in the United States at the end of the nineteenth century, at the same time that efforts were being made to standardize education for nurses and to establish specific criteria for nursing curricula. Today, formal nursing education programs generally may be categorized as basic or graduate level. Three major paths are available for an individual to obtain basic nursing education: diploma schools, associate degree programs, and baccalaureate degree programs. Regardless of the program, however, the rapid changes in the nursing knowledge base make providing information to students a continual challenge.

Diploma schools, supported by and affiliated with hospitals, are the oldest of the formalized nursing programs leading to licensure. Although generally acknowledged to provide the best clinical experience, due to their "on the job" nature, many of these programs have closed since the mid-1960s (Phillips, 1995). During that same period, the American Nurses Association and others formally proposed the baccalaureate degree as the minimal degree needed for entry into professional practice.

Two-year associate degree programs are most often found in community colleges. According to Price and Capers (1995), the curriculum of associate degree nursing "focuses on basic concepts and principles of nursing and on the technical aspects of delivering care to clients in acute health care settings" (p. 27) and is not usually designed to include leadership experiences; rather, it emphasizes technical nursing skills. The graduate receives an associate of arts degree.

Baccalaureate nursing education includes the general education required of all baccalaureate graduates, plus the scientific and clinical training necessary to assess care needs and to implement nursing care in a variety of settings; students also receive instruction on both nursing and management theory. Graduates receive a bachelor of science degree. Nurses with this type of education are expected to function in leadership roles.

Regardless of the type of education, all these graduates take the same licensure examination, and those who pass it become registered nurses (RNs).

According to the 1995 National League for Nursing (NLN) annual survey of RN programs (1996b), the number of both baccalaureate programs and associate degree programs has increased over the past 20 years, while the number of diploma programs has steadily decreased. As of January 1995, there were over 1,500 basic RN programs in the United States with over 250,000 students enrolled.

Graduate education consists of both master's and doctoral programs. The 1994 NLN Survey (National League for Nursing, 1996c) indicated that the number of master's programs had increased by 24, reaching a total of 276. Master's programs in nursing have traditionally emphasized three areas of focus: education, administration, and clinical practice. Two practice areas—nurse practitioner and advanced clinical practice—currently account for almost 90 percent of students enrolled at the master's level.

Advanced practice nursing includes nurse practitioners, nurse midwives, clinical nurse specialists, and nurse anesthetists. Graduate education for the latter two are included in the NLN category Advanced Clinical Practice Programs. These are specialty areas that may be more often associated with hospital and acute care, while nurse practitioners and nurse midwives are primary care providers who generally function under the supervision, direct or indirect, of a physician outside the hospital or in an acute care setting. The advanced clinical practice nurse functions as a mentor, teacher, researcher, and role model, as well as caregiver. This nurse is a resource both for other nurses as well as patients and their families. As such, it is essential that access is available to current information about their particular areas of practice as well as the profession as a whole.

Almost half of the more than 5,000 nurses enrolled in nurse practitioner programs have chosen family nurse practitioner programs. The nurse practitioner may function in health centers, hospitals, work sites, schools, clinics, and group practices in rural and urban settings. As nurses have recognized the potential opportunity that exists for an expanded role in the current health care delivery environment, with its emphasis on cost containment and managed care and its need for primary care providers, there has been a tremendous increase in enrollment in such programs.

The development of doctoral education in nursing has followed an interesting path. Initially, nurses received a doctoral education in fields other than nursing, which according to Meleis (1988), began with a doctorate in education from Columbia University in 1924. This was necessary to graduate a sufficient number (and critical mass) of nursing faculty in university programs—nurses who were able to both teach and administer nursing programs. At that time, the science of nursing itself was not thought to warrant its own academic degree program.

4

By 1962, however, the Nurse Scientist program, funded by federal grants, offered opportunities at 10 universities from which nurses could obtain PhD degrees in several fields including sociology, microbiology, psychology, and nursing, among others (Gortner, 1991). Since then, other nursing degrees offered include the Doctor of Nursing Science (DNS, DSN, DNSc) and the Doctor of Nursing (ND).

These degrees differ in their focus. The EdD program trains future administrators and faculty members (Gorney-Fadiman, 1981), while the PhD program aims to prepare nurses to teach, conduct research, and to practice, generally with an emphasis on the first two areas. The DNS programs focus more on clinical expertise than on conduct of research. Cleland (1976) described the nurse with a DNS degree as a utilizer of research rather than one who conducts the actual research.

The number of programs providing doctoral education for nurses has steadily increased over the last two to three decades, with accompanying increases in enrollment. In 1983, there were 33 such programs (National League for Nursing, 1996c); by 1992, this number had almost doubled.

Certification

In addition to basic and advanced educational preparation, nurses have received recognition through a variety of certification mechanisms for credentialing in a specialty or advanced practice area. Certification examinations are taken as a means of validating knowledge and competence for advanced or specialty practice. Although certification examinations have long been offered through specialty organizations, these examinations have never been standardized. Because of the many certification opportunities available (Fickeissen, 1990), the American Association of College of Nursing (AACN) has called for a uniform certification process, but until such a standard is in place, specialty organizations and individual states will continue to determine individual certification requirements. For example, the American Nurse Credentialing Center (ANCC), established by the American Nurses

Association in 1973, currently certifies nurses in at least 26 different areas. The ANCC certification categories include a generalist, who must be a registered nurse with several thousand hours of practice; a clinical nurse specialist and nurse practitioner, both of whom require a master's degree or higher in nursing along with other educational and practice prerequisites. Some specialty organization certifications are for those areas of practice for which there are no ANCC counterparts. Any uniform process would have to include all specialty certifications. Such a process would give the public-at-large the right to expect similar levels of performance from all advanced practice nurses.

Other Educational Formats

Three factors have prompted administrators of nursing schools to develop creative approaches to educational formats: the severe nursing shortage of the 1980s, the increased emphasis on baccalaureate education, and the number of professionals in other areas interested in the profession of nursing. Two such programs are the RN to BSN and the BA/BS (in other disciplines) to either BSN or MSN.

One institution that offers multiple programs is the Frances Payne Bolton School of Nursing at Case Western Reserve University in Cleveland, Ohio. It lists the following programs: Generic Baccalaureate, RN Baccalaureate, Accelerated RN Baccalaureate, BSN for Second Degree, MSN, MN for Nurses with Non-Nursing Degrees, MSN/MBA, Post-Master's ND, ND for Nurses with Non-Nursing Degrees, and PhD Degree.

In addition, alternative programs are being developed to provide education for nurses for whom there is little or no direct access to university programs or who are unable to attend classes on a regular basis. Distance education programs, one such alternative, may include classes conducted in a local hospital, in multiple sites across a large region, or via the Internet or television. Students enrolled in these programs must, however, have access to the resources and information offered in these nontraditional formats.

Specific programs of this type include the Distance Learning Program at California State University, Dominguez Hills, which utilizes various kinds of electronic delivery methods including compressed video and satellite to transmit its courses; and the Mind Extension University, a Colorado-based organization that connects courses from several universities or colleges including George Washington University and University of Colorado, Colorado Springs, with individuals at home or in an office. (Nursing is only one of the disciplines included in these programs, which pose the additional challenge of providing information resources for their students in the same manner as in the classroom.) California State University, Dominguez Hills, coordinates the Statewide Nursing Program in California that includes nursing classes given at local sites across the state, particularly in areas where this type of education might be otherwise difficult to obtain.

Levels of Practice

Implicit in the concept of practice *levels* is the hierarchical structure that historically has existed, and to some extent still exists, in hospital nursing practice. Traditionally, nurses functioned either in direct patient care, management, or educational roles. A registered nurse may have had several other registered nurses, licensed practical or vocational nurses, and nurses aides reporting to her or him, depending on the structure and philosophy of the facility. The recent trend toward managed care has resulted in a more horizontal structure that requires fewer registered nurses in hospitals, where direct patient care has often been shifted to a different type of health care worker: a care technician, aide, or other unlicensed staff member.

This horizontal continuum of care has expanded outside the acute care setting, generating an increased need for home health care and other nurses in different environments. Patients frequently leave the hospital still needing some degree of supervised nursing care; and the farther removed the patient is from the acute care setting, the greater his or her need for a nurse with independent clinical judgment, expertise, and education. The emphasis in nursing education and practice will shift to one of community-based care; that is, offered outside the acute care setting and focused not just on patient care but on disease prevention and health promotion as well, concepts that have been and continue to be of great interest to nursing.

Practice levels can also refer to the differences between degree achievement: whether associate, baccalaureate, or master's. As mentioned earlier, the debate in the profession continues over the level of education that should be required for entry into professional practice.

New Roles

The nursing environment is changing from moment to moment. Although De Tornyay (1993) reported that, in 1988, more than two-thirds of nurses practiced in hospitals, that is changing and will continue to change over the next decades. Today, there are few limitations on the roles that nurses can and do fill, from nurse attorneys to CEOs to members of Congress.

Further, the current economic environment and preponderance of managed care programs have generated the need for different settings for health care delivery, along with a different emphasis on its content. As noted previously, in the near future, nursing education will emphasize community-based practice and health promotion activities, which will be carried out in settings as diverse as the workplace, senior centers, hospices, day care centers, homeless shelters, and malls.

As more of these services are provided outside of acute care environments, more independent practice will evolve. And more independent practice potentially means greater utilization of advanced practice nurses. Many such nurses do not complete graduate programs in their specialty, but achieve their expertise through continuing education or experience and become certified by examination for advanced or specialty practice.

Another new care setting in which advanced practice nurses can participate is the nurse-managed center. The AACN Position Statement on Nursing's Agenda for the 21st Century (American Association of Colleges of Nursing, n.d.) includes recommendations for group faculty practice, joint appointments for faculty in both clinical and educational facilities, and practice collaboration with other disciplines. Nurse-managed centers can meet these recommendations.

Case manager is a new role for nurses, one that has evolved as a vital part of cost containment efforts on the part of both health maintenance organizations and acute care facilities. In the future, graduate schools will consider case management as a specialty because of the skills required and the independent nature of the practice.

Nursing informatics, too, will be recognized as a new specialty. Nurses practicing in this field will be expert not only at utilizing and manipulating data, but at acquiring it as well. As more nurses become more familiar with computers and the Internet, these information specialists will become important and in-demand resources.

Nurse attorney, another growing specialty, offers nurses the opportunity to participate in malpractice cases or to serve as legal consultants on health care issues. Consulting nurses also serve as telephone triage specialists, providing information to consumers who call with questions about symptoms, injuries, or the necessity to seek medical care.

The preceding are just a few of the many roles now available to nurses today, and the list will continue to grow as the expertise and capabilities of nurses become more widely recognized. A corresponding growth in information needs accompanies the expansion in the nursing profession, a topic covered in the next section.

PROVIDING INFORMATION RESOURCES AND SERVICES FOR NURSING

Nursing is an information-based profession, both from an education and practice perspective. Throughout a nurse's education and in practice, he or she must be able to adeptly access and assimilate information in order to maintain an up-to-date knowledge base (Weaver, 1993). This knowledge base is the cornerstone of an effective practitioner, regardless whether that practitioner is an administrator, educator, or clinician. Continual access to information resources is an essential component for ongoing professional development and competency. Information resources and services are usually developed to accommodate the type of institution and or role in which the nurse functions. Therefore, the guidelines and standards discussed in later chapters are generally modified to accommodate operations within a specific institutional environment. By way of introduction, the following are examples of some of the types and/or formats that information resources and services may take within individual institutions.

One-Person Library

In smaller institutions or institutions with limited information resources, a single person may be responsible for all phases of operations, from the acquisition of resources to their arrangement and dissemination. Depending on the needs of the institution, this person may even be only a part-time employee. While this type of arrangement affords the individual an increased sense of autonomy, information acquisition and dissemination are labor-intensive, so it is essential that the one-person library institute clearly defined policies and procedures to maximize the availability of all resources. Often, an information professional functioning in such a library will want to develop a peer network to enable an exchange of information and aid in problem solving.

Separate Library

In many institutions, collections related to specialty topics are maintained separately. This practice may be based on a variety of reasons ranging from the organization's mission to the physical configuration of buildings. For example, in a large university environment, a school of nursing may occupy an entire building that contains the library, media center, nursing laboratory, and classrooms. This arrangement facilitates more efficient communication and generally supports the development of expert subject information staff. However, because of the interdisciplinary nature of nursing and health care, this setup may force staff to constantly request nursing-related information from off-site sources. And although this physical arrangement may enable peer networking, the libraries may be understaffed since parent institutions have to maintain numerous separate institutional information resource centers and libraries.

Integrated Collections

Probably the most common type of library is the integrated collection. In this type of facility, all of an institution's library and information resources are centralized into one comprehensive service unit. Depending on the size of the institution, it may also contain departmental collections of materials, but overall, acquisition, cataloging, and the arrangement and access to collections are centralized. In some institutions, this has meant the integration of topically related items in different physical formats plus an array of hardware, software, and audiovisual equipment strategically located to maximize collection use. This arrangement gives users easy access to the broadest range of materials within one physical setting, and administratively, may be the most cost-effective approach to providing information resources and services.

Clinical Units

The manner in which nursing care is delivered and the need for quick access to disease and patient-related information has prompted a variety of approaches for accessing information at clinical units. The LATCH (literature attached to the chart) concept was an initiative developed to bring print literature related to a patient's condition to the unit and make it a part of the patient record (Stearns, Ottoson, & Haitz,1985). Some variations of the LATCH concept, such as the Patient Care-Related Readings (PCRR) were developed (Hutchinson, Malamud, Stearns, & Moulton, 1981).

In addition, some health care facilities have implemented the role of clinical librarian. Clinical librarians become part of the patient care team and provide information during daily reports or other patient-related conferences (Barbour & Young, 1986). For both the LATCH concept and clinical librarians, an intermediary is utilized to acquire and provide appropriate case-related information.

The trend today is to make health care providers information-literate and, in many cases, to provide the needed information resources where care occurs (Nurses, 1996). As the health care delivery system changes, it will become necessary to provide more clinical information services in freestanding clinical sites such as ambulatory surgery centers, diagnostic and treatment centers or public health clinics. In some cases, these may be provided as distance services.

Extension and Distance Services

Not all health providers have direct physical access to a library and/or information resources. This may be the result of inadequate financial resources to support services or of a specific decision on the part of an organization's administration. An example is a large health care network that contains two large acute care facilities, plus a series of affiliated but physically remote clinics or diagnostic centers. In this physical configuration, information services to the outlying clinics may be provided more cost-effectively by various methods such as circuit rider programs (Pifalo, 1994), telefacsimile networks for document delivery (Bergen & Barron, 1994), or video teleconferencing (Shomaker, 1995). As these technologies continue to develop, more institutions will be examining the issues of information access rather than collection maintenance.

Use of Evolving Technologies

The concept of a library without walls is not new, but never before has its potential been so imminent (Artis, 1994). How and what information is stored and transmitted over communication networks is evolving at an unparalleled rate. Basic print indexes have been replaced by computerized indexes, which are now globally available. More often, documents are readily available via computerized networks. Students can now access the full text of periodicals online, and interact with multimedia online environments such as the virtual hospital and the visible human project (Ackerman, 1995). From most locations, students and practitioners can take part in video conferences with experts from around the world. Already, access to the global array of information resources seems instant and unlimited, yet we are only at the beginning of this odyssey.

THE DEVELOPMENT OF LIBRARIES AND PROVISION OF INFORMATION RESOURCES AND SERVICES BY PROFESSIONAL AND SPECIALTY ORGANIZATIONS

For many years, Virginia Henderson, noted nurse theorist and promoter of libraries, called for the development of a National Library of Nursing, which would parallel the activities of the National Library of Medicine. She envisioned this library as a great repository of both historical and current materials, and as a comprehensive coordinated means of collecting the profession's literature. In this era of connectivity and fiscal restraint, however, it seems unlikely that such a library will ever be developed. Instead, nursing libraries and specialized information resources are evolving around specific institutional and/or association needs and missions. Specialized associations are one of the best information resources for publications, expert referral systems, and computerized information access (Eldredge, 1996). The following is a brief overview of some of the organizations that produce information products and have systems to provide information services to a specific segment of nursing clientele.

International Nursing Organizations

Within the international nursing community, three groups, the Canadian Nurses Association (CNA), the Royal College of Nursing

(RCN), and Sigma Theta Tau International, probably maintain the largest and most sophisticated collections of nursing information resources and services.

The Canadian Nurses Association. CNA's Helen K. Mussallem Library contains approximately 16,000 book and document titles and 600 periodical titles. The library also provides reference and research services and permits the loan of materials. It maintains a series of publications related to Canadian nursing research, the historical collections of the CNA, and a suggested reading list of periodicals for nurses.

The Royal College of Nursing. The RCN, with a membership base of over 300,000, is considered the world's largest professional nursing organization. Its multipurpose functions relate to three broad areas: labor relations, education, and professional issues (Friend, 1994). The College offers a wide array of services and publications, within which context is the division of Library and Information Service, the collection and library services support activities. In 1996, the College began to produce the library's journal database and full text of many of the collection's serial publications in CD-ROM format (T. Shepard, personal communication, October 1995).

Sigma Theta Tau International. Sigma Theta Tau, established in 1922, is the honor society of nursing. In the late 1980s, within the context of strategic planning efforts directed at nursing research, a major focus of the society, the organization set out to design and construct an international headquarters to house a world-class library. The library facility, eventually named after the aforementioned Virginia Henderson, was innovative both in content and its approach to provide access to the collection. Truly a library without walls or the usual print resource collection, it was designed as an electronic library containing a series of databases accessible via computer, and included such material as the first online nursing journal, *The Online Journal of Knowledge Synthesis for Nursing* (Killion, 1994). Contents and services of the Virginia Henderson Library continue to expand and are now accessible on the Internet.

National and State Nursing Organizations

Although a number of nursing organizations boast national membership, the majority relate to specialty practice, whereas the American Nurses Association and the National League for Nursing are considered the generalist multipurpose organizations for professional nursing. Within these organizations' structure are state-level groups, described in the following subsections.

American Nurses Association. The ANA, founded in 1896 as the Nurses' Associated Alumnae, is the national organization for registered professional nurses. Its members are the constituent state nurses associations (SNAs), and individual participation is enabled through membership in an SNA.

ANA produces a significant number of information products that are available for purchase (American Nurses Association, 1996). These products generally address broad policy issues, generic standards of clinical practice, and staff development and certification. Formats vary, ranging from small pamphlets, books, newsletters, and magazines to audiovisual materials. Following its corporate relocation to Washington, DC, in the early 1990s, ANA became increasingly aware of the need to develop a more comprehensive approach to information acquisition and utilization. The new corporate headquarters included a staff-only library and a records management facility, and ANA saw the need to provide a variety of online information services to its constituent SNA members. Subsequently, ANA developed ANA*NET (American Nurses Association, 1994), initially as a pilot project for the purpose of facilitating access by a limited number of state nurses associations to computerized communications, as well as full-text and bibliographic databases. The network now includes all state nurses associations, and databases have been expanded to include topics on health policy, legal developments, nursing issues and policy, economic and general welfare, salary and benefit information, and practice information. ANA is currently developing additional and Internet-accessible information resources for the general nursing community (ANA, 1996).

The National League for Nursing. Like the American Nurses Association, the National League for Nursing (NLN) is a broadly focused national nursing organization. Established in 1893 as the American Society of Superintendents of Training Schools for Nurses, unlike ANA, the NLN has a much broader membership base; it does not restrict its membership to registered nurses.

The NLN does not maintain a formal internal library for staff or members, but it is a significant producer of information resources for the profession of nursing, the majority of which are available through NLN Press. Many of the directory and statistical documents are produced by the League's Center for Research in Nursing Education and Community Health (Center for Research in Nursing Education, 1996), a useful source of information beyond its specific publications. Initially, NLN information products focused on nursing education, career development, and accreditation issues, but the League continues to steadily expand the scope of the topical coverage of its publications. Current resources cover the following areas: caring, informatics, contemporary theory and practice, gender studies, gerontology, history, health care reform, holistic health, and women's issues. Many of these areas contain information appropriate for utilization by health care consumers (National League for Nursing, 1996a). Presently, the League is considering providing electronic access to its vast array of print resources. Although the League has a structure that allows for state-level constituents, research did not indicate any specific information collections or services within it.

State Nurses Associations. As separately incorporated constituent members of ANA, state nurses associations vary greatly in size, which significantly impacts the types of information resources they produce and maintain. Generally, individual SNAs collect resources related to the practice environment for their particular states. In policy areas, they may also function as an information resource for the nonnursing community. Often, staff members are themselves the primary information resources of their associations.

In recent years, several SNAs have made an effort to more formally structure access to their information resources. Beyond their regular publication programs, they have created specialized libraries and/or online computerized information resources. For example, the New Hampshire Nurses Association has enabled access to its resources via a Web site (Schuman, 1995), and the Massachusetts Nurses Association and the Pennsylvania Nurses Association provide small specialized print collections with limited staff assistance to these materials. The most comprehensive SNA information provider, the New York State Nurses Association (NYSNA), maintains a collection of nearly 10,000 items and provides in-depth policy-related reference services to its staff and members. Information services are also available to nonaffiliated individuals on a fee-for-service basis. The NYSNA has recently installed computer equipment and software to institute a member-accessible bulletin board system that will eventually provide access to all the association's information resources.

Specialty Nursing Organizations

Specialty nursing organizations began to develop in the 1930s (Kelly, 1995). From 1950 to the 1970s, the number of specialty organizations rapidly increased to represent nearly every practice area (Jaszczak, 1996). This growth continues as the face of health delivery systems changes. Most specialty nursing organizations provide information resources within a publications program, and individuals who need topically specific information such as classification of nursing diagnosis, clinical practice standards, and guidelines would do well to start their research with requests to these specialty organizations. However, a limited number of these organizations do maintain additional resource collections and may provide some type of access to their collections. Following are a few of those organizations.

American Association of Critical-Care Nurses. AACN maintains a small library of materials, which are primarily staff and leadership resources. The collection functions as a repository of items produced by AACN. About 20 percent of the collection is from outside sources. The collection is not available for outside users, but individuals who consult professional staff at AACN for

17

assistance may have their questions answered in the form of documents from this collection.

The Association of Operating Room Nurses. AORN maintains the largest and most comprehensive collection of all the specialty nursing organizations. With a focus on perioperative nursing, the association's collection contains approximately 3,500 books and 350 journal subscriptions, as well as a selection of audiovisual materials. Although the primary clientele of the library are the association's staff and leaders, it does provide a variety of information services to members and other health care and business and industry professionals. General information about the library and AORN are available on the Internet at http://www.aorn.org.

Under Development. As organizations evolve, their needs for information also change. At present, two specialty nursing organizations—the Association of Women's Health, Obstetric, and Neonatal Nursing, and the Oncology Nursing Society—are developing library collections and systems for utilization of their information resources and services (K. DeGeorges, personal communication, October 15, 1996; D. Visconti, personal communication, October 18, 1996).

DEVELOPMENT OF NURSING LITERATURE

Nursing literature consists of many publications in different formats, and new forms are being developed continually. Currently the literature includes, but is not limited to, books, journals, textbooks, reference books, audiovisuals, software, pamphlets, position papers, practice guidelines, standards of practice, newsletters, and electronic documents.

Books and Journals. Books and journals, the oldest forms of nursing literature, began to be published in the United States soon after the advent of modern nursing. *A Manual of Nursing* from New York's Bellevue Training School and *A Handbook of Nursing for Family and General Use* from New Haven's Connecticut Training School both were published before 1880. These texts functioned "as valuable resources for both students and teachers, providing them with lessons in curriculum, etiquette, and nursing care" (Lippman, 1990). Other standard specialty textbooks such as *The Nursing Care of the Nervous and Insane,* published in 1898, were also available.

The nineteenth century saw the publication of the first nursing journals. According to Flaumenhaft and Flaumenhaft (1989), the first American nursing journal, *The Nightingale,* was published in 1886. Initially, journals were general in subject matter; for example, the *American Journal of Nursing, Nursing,* and *RN.* Specialty journals such as the *Journal of the American Association of Industrial Nurses* and *AORN Journal* began appearing in the 1950s and 1960s, as did *Nursing Research,* the goal of which was to keep nurses informed of current research, and, to encourage the conduct of such research.

Indexes to the Literature.   Many years after the development of the first journals, an index to the nursing literature was clearly necessary. The first to meet this need was the *Cumulative Index to Nursing Literature* (CINL). Printed in 1961 and covering literature for the period of 1956–1960, CINL focused on indexing 17 English serial titles. With the exception of the *American Association of Industrial Nurses Journal,* a specialty journal, the index focused on general coverage, although subsequent volumes reflected the growth in the nursing literature to include journals for surgical nurses, nurse anesthetists, nurse educators, cardiovascular nurses, geriatric nurses, other nursing specialties and allied health. CINL's extended coverage was reflected in its new name: the *Cumulative Index to Nursing & Allied Health Literature*™ (CINAHL).

A second printed nursing index, the *International Nursing Index*® (INI), published by the American Journal of Nursing Company in collaboration with the National Library of Medicine, began publication in 1966. It provided access to the journal literature in the United States as well as to the English and foreign language journals of nursing in other countries.

A third valuable index to the nursing literature is the *Nursing Studies Index,* first published in 1963 with the goal to recognize and index materials written between 1900–1959, and which were otherwise unindexed; produced in reverse chronological order, Volume IV covered the period 1957–1959, while Volume I, published in 1972, included the years 1900–1929. This "guide to reported studies, research in progress, research methods, and historical materials" (*Nursing Studies Index*, 1963, p. iii) was published by Lippincott under the direction of Virginia Henderson, the well-known nursing theorist.

Over the last two decades, the nursing literature has been enriched by the development of highly specialized journals such as *Cancer Nursing, Journal of Gerontological Nursing,* and *Journal of Nursing Administration.* The current health care environment has encouraged the publication of other journals such as *Computers in Nursing, Home Healthcare Nurse,* and *Holistic Nursing Practice.*

Electronic Age. As noted at the beginning of this chapter, electronic technology has and continues to have an effect on the access to nursing literature. Much of the literature previously mentioned is also available in electronic formats such as CD-ROM or on the Internet. The first nursing journal published specifically for online access is *The Online Journal of Knowledge Synthesis for Nursing,* launched in 1995 by Sigma Theta Tau International, the honorary nursing organization. Because it is published online, the journal staff is able to add new articles as they are produced rather than on a less-timely production schedule. Other journals developed for online delivery include: *Nursing Standard,* a Royal College of Nursing publication, which has an online component (*Nursing Standard Online*) that is accessible to Internet users; the *Australian Electronic Journal of Nursing Education*; and the *Online Journal of Issues in Nursing.* No doubt, many more will appear.

Indexes to the nursing literature have also been converted to electronic formats, which has made them faster to use, more effective, and very user-friendly. The ability to combine various indexing terms, for example, has significantly reduced the time it takes to conduct a literature search. Another advantage is that material such as abstracts, references, and full-text documents that would make a print publication far too expensive to produce can be included in their electronic counterparts.

Electronic publication of these journals and indexes is not without its challenges. Interesting and difficult questions have been raised regarding issues such as copyright, access to certain types of information and corresponding royalty payments, document delivery, and downloading and printing of electronically published journals. These questions await answers. And what of the "old" copies of these journals? Will they be maintained; and if so, where?

Limitations of Nursing Literature for Advanced Practice

Although nursing literature is a valuable source of information for various kinds of practice, in many cases, it will not, and should not, be the only body of literature referenced. For the advanced practice nurse, a category that includes nurse practitioners, nurse midwives, nurse anesthetists, and clinical nurse specialists, one particular body of literature will not be sufficient for obtaining adequate information, thus, advanced practice nurses should not limit themselves to only one type of literature for all questions. Just as the research question drives the design and methodology of a study, the practice question determines the literature that should be consulted. Psychological, sociological, business, and hospital literature are just a few of the other possible resources in which nurses should be interested. The databases that index these types of literature can be used to locate these alternative resources useful to nurses. Examples of these databases include ERIC® for educational materials, PsychLit® for psychological literature, Social SciSearch® for sociological literature, ABI/INFORM™ for business literature, or HealthSTAR for hospital literature. (Additional databases of interest to nurses are discussed in other chapters of this book.)

The Future of Literature and Information Resources for the Nursing Profession

One of the goals of this chapter has been to point out the many changes occurring in the nursing environment that will affect future needs of its professionals. Continual advances in computer technology, resulting in ever more sophisticated and complex equipment, will require nurses in all areas to be computer literate as well as current in the literature. Certainly, the new generation of nurses, who have been exposed to computers throughout their education, will be more comfortable with this technology, and will expect easy access to it.

Computers that serve as both information resources as well as charting or record-keeping tools will be essential in the workplace. Electronic resources available at the patient's bedside will also become more commonplace. Home access via computer to indexes to the literature will also be necessary. As nurses become aware of the vast amounts of literature and information available, demands for these "fugitive" materials will increase. And as greater numbers of nurses seek baccalaureate and graduate degrees while continuing to work, many of them will utilize distance learning programs and will need to access libraries and other information resources via computer. The Internet is becoming an excellent resource for nurses seeking this type of information and service, patient education materials, and government documents. Internet special interest groups and listservs are also available for consultation and communication. Further, nursing organizations are placing bulletin boards and forums on their World Wide Web sites to encourage conversations between nurses all over the world. These, too, are excellent sources for information.

As more nurses produce excellent research that is being published widely, resources such as Sigma Theta Tau's Virginia Henderson Library and its Research Directory will become widely used. Such resources will enable access to information about ongoing and completed research that may not be available elsewhere.

While the demands for greater information access increase, the changing nature of the work environment—resulting in a shift into community settings such as home health and parish nursing—will take nurses farther away from standard library facilities available in the hospital or academic setting. They will need to be able to download materials from Internet sites and to have access to various other methods of document delivery.

Nursing students at all levels must be encouraged to update their knowledge through the literature throughout their careers. Without question, computer literacy is the key to these resources, and will remove the barriers to resources that existed in the past.

CONCLUSION

Although this chapter has focused on access to information resources as crucial for the practice and education of nurses, the human component in this effort must be addressed as well. The services of both the experienced librarian and the experienced educator are essential to assist nurses to locate and properly use resources. Similarly, educators must demand that students develop habits of synthesizing and applying the resources to their practice environments. As Weaver (1993) points out, "the librarian and instructor must work together" (p. 31) to accomplish the ultimate goal of information literacy.

REFERENCES

Ackerman, M. (1995). The visible human project. *Interactive Healthcare Newsletter, 11*(7/8), 1.

American Association of Colleges of Nursing. (n.d.). *Position statement. The baccalaureate degree in nursing as minimal preparation for professional practice.* Washington, DC: Author.

American Nurses Association. (1994). *ANA*NET user guide: The future of nursing requires instantaneous access to information.* Washington, DC: Author.

American Nurses Association. (1996). *American nurses publishing catalog, 1996.* Washington, DC: Author.

ANA launches site on the World Wide Web. (1996). *The American Nurse, 28*(4), 25.

Artis, S. (1994). *Library without walls: Plug in and go.* Washington, DC: Special Libraries Association.

Axley, S. (1996). *Communication at work.* Westport, CT: Greenwood Press.

Barbour, G. L., & Young, M. N. (1986). Morning report: Role of the clinical librarian. *Journal of the American Medical Association, 255*, 1921–1922.

Bergen, L., & Barron, M. M. (1994). The use of facsimile (fax) machines to transmit medical information. *Journal of the American Health Information Management Association, 65*(9), 60–62.

Center for Research in Nursing Education & Community Health. (1996). *Nursing data review, 1996.* New York: National League for Nursing.

Cleland, V. (1976). Developing a doctoral program. *Nursing Outlook, 24,* 631–635.

DeTornyay, R. (1993). Nursing education: Staying on track. *Nursing & Health Care, 14,* 302–306.

Eldredge, J. D. (1996). Associations that produce significant publications for the health sciences: Results from tracking a phantom literature. *Bulletin of the Medical Library Association, 84,* 572–579.

Fickeissen, J. L. (1990). 56 ways to get certified. *American Journal of Nursing, 90,* 50–57.

Flaumenhaft, E., & Flaumenhaft, C. (1989). American nursing's first textbooks. *Nursing Outlook, 37,* 185–188.

Friend, B. (1994). Going strong: Royal College of Nursing. *Nursing Times, 90*(8), 48.

Gorney-Fadiman, M. J. (1981). A student's perspective on the doctoral dilemma. *Nursing Outlook, 29,* 650–654.

Gortner, S. R. (1991). Historical development of doctoral programs: Shaping our expectations. *Journal of Professional Nursing, 7,* 45–53.

Hutchinson, S., Malamud, J., Stearns, N. S., & Moulton, B. (1981). Preselected literature for routine delivery to physicians in a community hospital based patient care related program. *Bulletin of the Medical Library Association, 69,* 236–239.

Jaszczak, S. (Ed.). (1996). *Encyclopedia of associations* (31st ed.). Detroit, MI: Gale Research.

Kelly, L. Y. (1995). *Dimensions of professional nursing* (7th ed.). New York: McGraw-Hill.

Killion, V. J. (1994). Information resources for nursing research: The Sigma Theta Tau International electronic library and online journal. *Medical References Services Quarterly, 133,* 1–17.

Lippman, D. T. (1990). Early nursing textbooks. *Imprint, 37,* 109–110, 112.

Meleis, A. I. (1988). Doctoral education in nursing: Its present and its future. *Journal of Professional Nursing, 4,* 436–446.

Monsen, R. B. (1996). Our finest hour may have arrived . . . threats to nursing as a profession and as a discipline. *Journal of Pediatric Nursing: Nursing Care of Children and Families, 11,* 81.

National League for Nursing. (1996a). *National League for Nursing 1996–1997 book catalog.* New York: Author.

National League for Nursing. (1996b). *Nursing datasource 1996: Vol. 1. Trends in contemporary RN nursing education.* New York: Author.

Introduction: Information Resources and Services

National League for Nursing. (1996c). *Nursing datasource 1996: Vol. 2. Graduate education in nursing: advanced practice nursing.* New York: Author.

Nurses and their computers: Clinical innovators. (1996). *Sigma Theta Tau International Reflections, 22*(2), 8–30.

Nursing studies index. (1963). Philadelphia: Lippincott.

Phillips, M. K. (1995). The future of diploma programs. *Imprint, 42*(2), 56–57.

Pifalo, V. (1994). Outreach to health professionals in rural area. *Medical Reference Services Quarterly, 13*(3), 19–26.

Price, C. R., & Capers, E. S. (1995). Associate degree nursing education: Challenging premonitions with resourcefulness. *Nursing Forum, 30,* 26–30.

Rush, S. L. (1992). Nursing education in the United States, 1898–1910: A time of auspicious beginnings. *Journal of Nursing Education, 31,* 409–414.

Schuman, A. J. (1995). Med Nexus brings the New Hampshire Nurses Association to the Internet. *Nursing News, 45*(6), 5.

Shomaker, D. (1995). WSRN state of the science papers. Research in nursing distance education: Defining the elephant. *Communicating Nursing Research, 28,* 133–145.

Stearns, N. S., Ottoson, J. M., & Haitz, M. C. (1985). Literature to go . . . Packets of selected articles which are attached to the charts of patients. *American Journal of Nursing, 85,* 1161–1162.

Weaver, S. M. (1993). Information literacy: Educating for life long learning. *Nurse Educator, 18,* 30–32.

SUGGESTED READINGS

Arnold, J. M., & Pearson, G. A. (Eds.). (1992). *Computer applications in nursing education and practice.* New York: National League for Nursing.

Blythe, J., Royle, J. A., Oolup, P., Potvin, C., & Smith, S. D. (1995). Linking the professional literature to nursing practice: Challenges and opportunities. *AAOHN Journal, 43,* 342–345.

Buckholtz, T. J. (1995). *Information proficiency: Your key to the information age.* New York: Van Nostrand Reinhold.

Johnson, M. B. (1990). The holistic paradigm in nursing: The diffusion of an innovation. *Research in Nursing & Health, 13,* 129–139.

Lang, N. M. (Ed.). (1995). *An emerging framework: Data system advances for clinical nursing practice.* Washington, DC: American Nurses Publishing.

Nurses and their computers: Clinical innovators. (1996). *Sigma Theta Tau International Reflections, 22*(2), 8–30.

Packard, S. A., Polifroni, C., & Shah, H. S. (1994). Rules and regulations governing nursing education. *Journal of Professional Nursing, 10*(2), 97–104.

Special Libraries Association. (1996). *Information revolution: Pathway to the 21st century.* Washington, DC: Author.

2

Basic Considerations in Administration: Resources, Services, and Accreditation

Caroline E. Mann, MSLS
Richard Barry, MLS
Deborah L. Graham, MLS

The nursing library is unique among those classified as special. Rarely a stand-alone entity, frequently a nursing collection is associated with a school of nursing, is part of a library system within an academic setting, or is a section of the hospital staff library. As with other specialized information collections, a nursing information resource center has to be adapted specifically to suit its environment, thus information in this chapter should be interpreted appropriately.

Administrative considerations in developing and managing information resources for nursing covered in this chapter focus on resources and services in relation to the parent organization, issues relating to the provision of services, library facilities and equipment, copyright, the Americans with Disabilities Act, the Library Bill of Rights, and library standards and accreditation.

RESOURCES AND SERVICES

Relationship to the Mission of the Parent or Sponsoring Institution

Library services are part of the overall objectives of the primary institution, and the interaction among all of the components of the institution is important. The library director needs to be clear about the structural levels within the organization and to whom the library staff reports. It is always most desirable that the director's position be at the administrative level of the institution. When the library director is part of the administrative team, the stage is set for the library to be managed as an autonomous entity rather than as a subdivision of some other department. The director can then exercise a certain level of authority regarding control over the responsibilities of library services (Darling, Bishop, & Colaianni, 1982). The library is accountable to the parent organization, not only for the resources provided by the institution, but for fulfilling and maintaining the institution's goals and objectives. These elements of responsibility, authority, and accountability can be delineated in an organizational chart of the institution, which serves to clarify the role of the library within the institution.

The institution's overall organizational structure may be centralized or decentralized. When the nursing library is a subspecialty (as in an academic library system) in a centralized system, it is a line item of the bigger picture. It competes with other departments and facilities for resources. In a decentralized system, the nursing library would have a more independent situation. The library director or manager would be operating a more or less independent operation, not one in direct competition with other similar departments.

The differences between a nursing collection as a separate entity versus as a subgroup of a larger institutional collection are important to review. A separate nursing collection's advantage is that it allows for direct control of the budget and operations, thereby reducing administrative reporting structures. A disadvantage is that a separate collection requires sufficient staff to maintain the collection and services.

In contrast, an integrated nursing collection would be housed with the larger health sciences collection and follow the policies and procedures of the larger collection. An example is a hospital setting where many specialty-practice libraries are integrated to form the main collection; no one predominates, and each reflects a practice area of the hospital. If the collection is part of a health sciences collection, then the nursing materials will become interspersed among other disciplines. It is also possible that the collection may be in various locations, such as undergraduate, graduate, or historical collections. The configuration of the hospital system may also influence the location of specific specialties within the nursing field.

The makeup of nursing libraries must also take into consideration that many nursing students are not enrolled in traditional on-campus programs, but rather matriculate in external degree programs, whose courses are offered in extended campus facilities in rural or inner-city areas. This raises questions regarding what to include in the various on-site and off-site collections, and which resources will be available through interlibrary loan, resource sharing, or commercial vendors. The answers to these questions depend upon the particular institutional goals, mission, and allocated resources. Therefore, it is vital that an in-depth analysis of policies relating to the extent of projected extension and distant services be examined to determine whether sufficient resources exist to provide the services in question.

A recent factor in maintaining adequate library services is that more institutions now offer services to "virtual" patrons, those connected to the institution electronically. Adequate equipment, such as computers, copiers, fax machines, and printers, must be provided to sustain these services. Further, policies on computer license agreements—regarding users and where they are located— have to be evaluated. For example, some programs do not allow dial-in access if they are loaded on a local area network (LAN); they are restricted to on-site use only.

Finally, interlibrary loan and document delivery are two other very important elements to consider when formulating policies for extension and distance services. But whatever the type of library system, it will need a clear and definitive mission statement with written policies to function effectively.

Policies and Procedures. Policies provide an overarching framework that delineates the role the library fulfills for the institution, therefore they must be rooted in a firm understanding of the goals of the parent institution. Depending upon the overall structure of the setting, the administration of the institution may wish to promulgate the policies. Procedures are the concrete actions the library follows in meeting the policies. For example, assume a library policy states that only members of the institution such as staff or students may use the library. A logical procedure then would be that the library staff should ask for identification of persons entering the library. In short, procedures should be based on established policy.

The elements to consider when creating policy and procedure revolve around the clientele: their needs, how to meet those needs, alternative possibilities, and the existing political and social context. The client may be determined by the parent institution or by the library director. The determination of who will be served by the library is important for planning the dispersion of resources and the management of personnel (Darling et al., 1982), because the clientele's needs for products, resources, and services will not be static, but will fluctuate and change over time. Certain core or basic requirements will be long-standing, but will be coupled with secondary needs of a temporary nature.

Once the client group and its associated needs are identified, it is necessary to analyze how best to meet these needs through technology, personnel, and budget. These elements should be evaluated annually in order to maximize the resources allocated to the library. Established policies and procedures provide a framework within which to operate in the present and to navigate to the future. Policy helps to determine when demands come from outside clientele, or when primary clientele demand services outside the scope of what the library can realistically offer. One goal should be to communicate library policies and services to the primary clientele, in order to make it clear to them that they are a select group, so as to raise their level of appreciation. Likewise, procedures should be spelled

30

out for various functions to establish an environment of consistency for the client. This will result in fewer areas needing close supervision and management. The long-term benefit of written policies and procedures is that all staff know and share the responsibilities of library functions. Staff then has at hand important information regarding operational issues such as the selection of materials, facilities, personnel needs for various duties, and the multiple types of service provided.

A written policy regarding the donation of books, journals, equipment, and audiovisual materials should also be established. A clear definition of the content of the collection will ensure that a substantial donation in one subject area will not require more space than was designed for it. Policy should also incorporate the library's involvement in outreach activities, training or instruction classes, library displays, institutional special events, grant activities, and fund-raising efforts.

Libraries are expensive propositions that often must operate on very tight and limited budgets. Fee for service is one option for recouping some of the expenses. Thus, assessing the institutional policy pertaining to collecting fees for services is important, along with the accounting and charge-back activities associated with collecting fees. Just determining fees can be a challenge, since the goal is not to make a profit but to recoup the costs of providing the service. Some services, including database searching, interlibrary loan, photocopying, and document delivery, have established costs and pricing, which should be calculated when formulating fee policy statements.

Policy that must be carried out by staff is best created as a participatory activity. Directives handed down from above without staff input will ultimately prove ineffective, or worse, be ignored. Top-down authoritarian management does not recognize nor respect the education and training of the staff. The most effective policy results from a bottom-up collaboration involving all staff responsible for administering that policy. With a large personnel pool, one approach is to assign various committees to work on specific issues, collecting all the relevant information into a workable, realistic, observable, and attainable policy or procedure. Another option is to have the librarian and library committee develop policies.

Library Committee. The library committee serves a very useful advisory capacity for the librarian. Composed of individuals who represent key or major groups of library clients, they are intermediaries who express the concerns and needs of the group they represent. Ideally, the library committee should represent a cross-section of the users. In addition, the library policies and procedures manual should outline the function of the committee to eliminate unnecessary confusion and conflict. It is important that the committee is consulted in a manner that assures no practice area is inadequately served. However, the librarian should be careful not to rely too heavily upon the committee and thus unconsciously surrender authority to the group.

One function of members of the committee might be to serve in an oversight capacity for specific areas of the library's responsibilities or for special projects. The committee can offer specific advice regarding such areas as research; practice specialties; and computer, electronic, CD, or Internet capabilities. The world of nursing is vast and specialized, with many new resources being developed daily, and the committee should be relied on to channel these emerging trends and issues to the librarian. The role of the library committee is to suggest, review, and revise policy; to provide important grassroots input and support for library procedures; and to provide a balanced perspective of any institutional situation. For those librarians who find themselves as the only library professional, such a committee offers important support in the institutional community for establishing programs, policies, and decisions.

Strategic Planning. The successful operation of a library requires keeping an eye on the future. A library director can begin to plot future direction through strategic planning. "Strategic planning is a process whereby managers establish an organization's long-term direction, set specific performance objectives, develop strategies to achieve these objectives in light of all the relevant internal and external circumstances, and execute the chosen action plans" (Moore & Vincent, 1994). This type of planning needs to be a collaborative effort involving all departments and personnel intimately involved with the nursing library, such as the hospital administration or the academic dean, who will contribute to the desired goals. The strategic plan should define clear responsibilities for objectives, and be integrated with the budgeting process. A manageable number of objectives realistic for the time period should be specified in clear and easily understood language. Departments and/or individuals, too, can develop long- and short-term objectives that support, develop, and advance the strategic plan of the institution.

There are four components to developing a strategic plan (Darling et al., 1982). Defining the mission and knowing the primary business of the organization is the starting point. This involves understanding the overall mission of the parent organization as it relates to the specific mission of the nursing library to determine how they complement one another. The second step is to define the optimal position for the library at some specific date, with accompanying goals and objectives. This ensures that organizations and institutions keep up with changing trends and technologies. Once the trends have been analyzed and a target has been established, the third element is to devise a plan or program to reach the target objective. The program is usually a multiphase, multiyear blueprint filled with short-range goals and objectives that lead to the long-range objective.

In addition to the preceding four steps, it is important to identify alternative strategies that enable quick responses to unanticipated changes in the context or environment. Doing so enables library staff to successfully readdress or reconfigure a short-range goal, or even the long-range plan.

Facilities and Equipment

Location. Any plan for the location of a library must take into consideration easy access for the greatest number of targeted clients. The Americans with Disabilities Act (ADA) requires access ramps, barrier-free entrance areas, automatic doors, and an elevator if necessary.

A second factor is the weight of the collection, which often prompts planners to place the library on the lowest level of a

building, which may or may not be ideal. If such a location is regarded by patrons as "out of the way," planning has not been successful. On the other hand, if the lowest level is also the entry level,
and patrons must pass the library to access the rest of the building,
the goal of being in a high-traffic location has been met. This would
also mean an elevator would be unnecessary for library access.

A central location should be sought when the institutional
offices or classrooms are in various buildings, although a less-
than-ideal location can be circumvented by the use of a LAN
that gives access to library databases via computer. This can be
coupled with a campus delivery service if there is sufficient staff
to fulfill requests.

Americans with Disabilities Act (Public Law 101-366). It is
impossible to know the physical capabilities of all library patrons.
Therefore, during the planning stages, adequate attention must be
paid to fire safety and air quality, and the potential for flood and
storm damage.

As already briefly mentioned, planning must take into account
the requirements of the Americans with Disabilities Act. More
specifically, the free flow of foot and wheel traffic around and between immovable objects in the library requires 36 to 42 inches of
space to conform to the law. Table heights and space should accommodate working comfortably from a wheelchair. Such patrons
must also have access to shelved materials; or sufficient staff should
be on hand to assist them. Patrons with disabilities have a varying
range of abilities, so it is appropriate to ask what assistance, if any,
is necessary.

An issue related to barrier-free access is what is known as assistive technology (Mates, 1992), tools, devices, or technologies
that make it possible for those with disabilities to use library resources. Some examples are telecommunications devices for the
deaf (TDDs), video display terminal (VDT) magnifiers, tactile
key indicators, large-print keyboards, magnifier/halogen lights,
and speech input computers (Mates, 1992, p. 21).

Space Planning. In addition to meeting ADA requirements,
the architect must address building codes specific to the particular

state and county. Planning a library space today requires that it be flexible functionally; that is, modular. Many business settings have a physical environment that is easily adaptable to changes within the organization. This concept is now applied to the library, where the emphasis is on adapting the space to meet the current needs of patrons. Open, airy, welcoming spaces will encourage more use than stuffy, poorly lighted, and drafty rooms.

Two major influences on the design and selection of furniture, shelving, and study carrels are ergonomics (the study of physiology) and the Americans with Disabilities Act. Both have precipitated the design and availability of furnishings that offer easy access and convenience. Purchasing library furniture made of good solid materials that will withstand years of use and abuse is always a good investment; and at the least, it should meet Business and Institutional Furniture Manufacturers Association (BIFMA) and American National Standards Institute (ANSI) standards for construction and durability. Some analysis will be necessary to determine the number of patrons using the library space at any one time, and to what extent it may need to accommodate other departments or functions.

Shelving space calculations should factor in 5 to 10 years of expansion in the collection. Usually, for the most visible areas, shelving material is of wood and metal for the rest. (Wood shelving is about 30 percent more expensive than the steel-bracket type, has height- and weight bearing limitations, and is not as fire-retardant.) Depending on the situation, compact shelving, which moves either by motor or manually along tracks in the floor, may be an option, especially when space is limited. But note that compact shelving requires flooring that bears weight at least two and a half to three times greater than that required by regular shelving.

Shelving needs are calculated on a shelf two-thirds full, with 16 the average number of volumes per shelf. A barrier-free space of 36 to 42 inches should be included between aisles, stacks, immovable furniture, and other objects to conform with the American with Disabilities Act. (For additional information on selecting shelving, refer to the "Storage Furniture" section in Chapter 8, Preservation.)

Environmental Controls. The library environment includes air-conditioning and lighting, and planning for adequate fresh air circulation coupled with appropriate levels of humidity, heat, and cooling requires expert advice. In spite of the increase in virtual access to library facilities, many clients still work on-site, and their physical needs must be met in accordance with established standards and codes. The impact of environmental phenomena, such as air pollution, should be taken into consideration when planning the facility. This means the building should have adequate safeguards to prevent it from becoming a "sick building." Materials, too, must be protected. Humidity control is important for preservation of materials; a relative humidity of 50 percent is recommended. This, combined with sufficient zone controls on air-conditioning equipment, should provide patrons with a pleasant atmosphere and ensure a long life for the collection.

Security. The security of the building or library space must not be overlooked. Even those libraries that operate on the honor system should take appropriate measures to ensure proper use of the facilities and the collection. Magnetic strips that work with scanning systems located at the doors can be inserted into the binding of books. An alarm sounds when a book has not been "demagnetized" upon checkout. This is the most popular system for monitoring clients exiting the library, but note that no system is foolproof.

Any staff members who need to work alone or in isolated areas of the building must be made to feel secure, because libraries are not immune to individuals wishing to do bodily harm. Thus, monitoring systems must be incorporated when planning the design of all entryways.

Safety. Closely related to security issues are accommodations for natural disasters, fire, and other accidental occurrences. The correct fire alarm and extinguishing systems should be installed so as to protect patrons and staff, yet not cause major damage to the collection or equipment when invoked. Any geographic area prone to natural disasters must consider their likelihood when planning the building in general and the shelving in particular. Local building codes provide adequate direction in planning for these contingencies.

Workstations.   Any location, whether counter, desk, or table, where people spend extended periods of time working can be considered a workstation. Individuals of various sizes and physical capabilities will be accessing these spaces, so it is ideal to have the ability to adjust the height of both the work surface and the seating. At least two online reference catalogs should be made available: one on a surface 38 inches high for standing access, and the other a wheelchair-accessible workstation, of standard seating height and adequate knee clearance. The monitors should be at least 15 inches or larger to accommodate users with low vision; or their design should enable the magnification or vocalization of information. Most reading and writing tasks should be performed at a height of about 28 inches, or at a height that enables patrons to keep their elbows bent at 90 degrees, with the wrists straight. Space for knees under work surfaces should be at least 30 inches wide with a depth of 19 inches and a height of 27 inches (Michaels & Michaels, 1992).

Lighting should be of a nonglare type that focuses on the task, rather than on any equipment screen that is already lighted. Work surface areas need rounded edges for comfort, and should be of a medium to light color to reduce contrast with text pages. Computer and electrical cables should be routed to the back of the workstation to prevent tampering, tripping, and entanglement in hands and feet. Workstations need at least six electrical outlets on different electrical circuits from the electronic equipment. Staff and patrons should be able to sit comfortably approximately 30 inches from any video display terminal.

CD-ROM Setups.   The advances and developments in this area of technology preclude making specific product identifications here, therefore it is important to consider all aspects of using this technology before making a decision about a specific approach. Remember that users will be accessing information from work, home, school, and while traveling, requiring simultaneous multiuser and multilocation access to multiple databases. To date, no singular alternative emerges as superior to any other. The system of choice will be determined largely by the systems currently in place at the institution, the level of support available for that technology, and available funds. System integration and industry standards are the cornerstones of planning and operation in this area, although novel approaches will emerge according to the capabilities and expertise of the technology consultants.

The librarian should establish a framework based on all the options for delivering information in the library or institution. Consideration should be given to variable costs of print, online, and CD products, both initially and over time. The licensing agreement that accompanies electronic software should be examined to determine whether any restrictions (on who is legally allowed to access it, how many users may access it simultaneously, and how often the agreement must be renewed) will affect library patrons (Cibbarelli, Gertel, & Kratzert, 1993).

If it is determined that the CD-ROM format is the most effective means for accessing information, the next step is to determine which configuration will best serve the needs of the client: a stand-alone system, network, jukebox, or file server. A stand-alone system should be evaluated from a practical point of view: Is it dictated by the library location, patron needs, and cable installation requirements? A small client population may be adequately served by this level of technology as opposed to one more complex, expensive, and requiring a higher level of technical support. The introduction of a stand-alone system may become the first step toward upward migration to a local area network (LAN)-based system. While stand-alone systems initially are financially more affordable, when viewed over the long term, the variable costs are higher than the total operating costs of a LAN-based system (Wilkinson, 1992).

Networking CD-ROM operations via a LAN is becoming increasingly popular as hardware and software costs decrease and technological sophistication increases. CD-ROM servers provide a wide range of options for memory, drive capacity, and processor speed. These servers can be configured for Ethernet, token-ring, ARCnet, or LANtastic networks as part of a Windows environment. Conversely, due to technology difficulties, the use of jukeboxs for CD-ROM has decreased. There are many network solutions available for system operation, one of which is the CD-ROM tower for multiuser access, which is becoming increasingly popular. And thanks to the steadily decreasing cost of CD-ROM drives, each application may now have its own drive, instead of having to share one in a jukebox environment. CD uniformity is important for achieving ease of use and successful retrieval by patrons. Windows environments often provide online tutorials that explain variations between applications, but most patrons prefer a more transparent system.

Remote access can be provided through a wide area network (WAN), accomplished by installing a gateway (which interconnects various devices running different communications protocols or operating systems) between the WAN and the LAN; or the CD-ROM drives can be installed directly to the WAN (Ka-Neg, 1992).

LAN Architecture. This discussion of LAN architecture centers on the two currently most popular systems: peer-to-peer, and file server. Peer-to-peer architecture is appropriate for those systems with fewer than 10 workstations; any more will reduce the speed of applications across the board. The positive side of peer-to-peer systems is that information can reside on any machine on the system, enabling complete communication among all machines. Peer-to-peer architecture is also cost effective. Programs such as Microsoft Workgroup for Windows and Windows 95 have the architecture built into the program; thus, setting up and running the LAN is relatively simple compared to a file server. The negative aspects of this system are management of the configuration and security. Because there are multiple sites, rather than a singular site for information and applications, getting a complete picture requires collecting all lists and directories. Security is difficult because the system is designed to be open, where users freely share information. The best security is password protection of files or applications.

A file server LAN architecture employs a single machine on which shared files and programs provide the basic components. This "dedicated" machine is the primary source for all applications; and each machine on the LAN communicates with the file server for applications. Based upon the configuration (memory, RAM, processor speed) of the dedicated file server, multiple workstations can be tied into it. The file server becomes the hub for all of the applications and programs on the LAN. A file server LAN should be used in conjunction with a graphical user interface (GUI) system to minimize training and help desk questions.

A file server obviously is easier to manage and upgrade: It is one server as compared to several in the peer-to-peer architecture. All of the applications and programs are in one machine, so troubleshooting, file maintenance, and system configuration can be accomplished from a centralized location. Upgrading a file server's memory or programs is easier with the dedicated machine, although it does require the system to be down for a period of time; but if clients are warned ahead of time and the upgrade is scheduled during off-peak usage periods, this can be accomplished with minimal inconvenience.

The disadvantages of a file server system are the cost and the need for a special operating system. A file server requires a large investment in a dedicated machine, powerful enough to run multiple applications simultaneously. Depending upon the number of stations and the type of applications running, huge amounts of memory can be taken up just in running the programs. Sufficient backup systems also have to be in place. And, because the file server LAN is built from the dedicated machine out to the others, a special operating system software is needed to enable the machines to interface and share applications and files. The Novell network is one of the most popular systems, but there are many others to choose from on the market.

LAN architecture also requires a consideration of wiring schemes. The cheapest and easiest to implement is an Ethernet, especially for small to medium-size systems. There are two types: thin net and 10-base-T. The thin net is a coaxial cable that is inexpensive to set up and run through the building. Its shortcoming is that if a break occurs anywhere on the system, the whole system shuts down. And such a break can occur when the connections are not tight or secure, the cable is pulled too taut, or it comes in contact with animals or water. The 10-base-T cable is basically telephone wire, and is less expensive, but it requires hubs (electronic repeaters and signal intensifiers) on the system. On the positive side, a break in this system generally does not shut down the entire system.

ARCnet is a third wiring scheme that has been available for a number of years. However, its low-performance capability does not make a good choice for modern applications. A fourth option, the token-ring scheme, has the same general layout as the 10-base-T, but token-ring gives much better performance. Unfortunately, its components are much more expensive. One other scheme, which is becoming more cost-effective and popular, is the 100-base-T, which operates at 10 times the speed of the 10-base-T.

When determining which wiring schemes to choose, the distance between machines and/or hubs will be an important factor. Distance limitations are caused by the resistance inherent in the cable, and vary according to the type of system. The maximum distance for Ethernet and 10-base-T is about 1,500 feet; for the token-ring, the maximum distance is about 3,000 feet. Broadband cable is likely to return to use in computer applications because of the scope of traffic it can handle. Now that video and JAVA are part of many applications, this wider band width will support these with greater efficiency.

The application of LAN architecture will be unique to each library situation. The variety of available hardware and software makes the combinations almost mind-boggling. To help in this regard, several of the large networks that supply company catalogs include schematic pictures of all of the possible LAN architectures. It is advisable to survey the possibilities for selecting a system that will grow and change along with the technological advances of science and the needs of your patrons.

Electronic Resources and Services.   Computers have become an integral part of libraries. In order to meet user needs, the library must provide access to the various types of electronic information resources available, including online bibliographic databases and the newly emerging Internet information resources.

Computer-searchable bibliographic databases are available in a number of forms but CD-ROM subscriptions (also available for books, journals, and many government documents) may be the most economical and provide sufficient access for smaller libraries. The advantage to these systems is that they are located on the library's computer or a local CD-ROM network and priced according to the number of users who can access the system at one time. Larger libraries may require a larger number of simultaneous user "ports," and can negotiate with vendors to have the desired databases mounted on the library's main computer. Which brings up an important task: choosing a database provider. Before doing so, be sure to obtain references, then check on how helpful they have been to established clients who have experienced problems in loading or troubleshooting either hardware or software. And ask about other services. Some vendors offer on-site training or a 24-hour help desk. Also consider how complex or easy the user interface is. For help in this endeavor, consult the professional library literature, where database providers are reviewed. A well-supported though more costly software package may be more cost-effective in the long run than a poorly supported system at a lower price. As users become accustomed to the availability of online search systems, the reliability of those systems reflects directly on the library, not the vendor, and can result in a positive, or devastating, effect on the library's reputation.

Another element to consider before adding CD-format materials to a library collection is that their usefulness is dependent on reliable computer equipment, and that users may require more personnel time than was necessary for print materials. Consequently, it may be more appropriate and considerate to locate equipment in an area where the noise inherent in user instruction will not disturb others.

The Internet, a high-speed electronic communication network that links all types of computers and terminals throughout the world is the most recent electronic resource, and one that is experiencing unparalleled growth. Standard electronic communications protocols allow rapid transmission of data (text, audio, and images) between sites. Within this network, computers that serve primarily as suppliers of information are called *servers*. A server might contain bibliographic databases that can be searched to find citations to articles in professional journals; or it might house a library of images dealing with a specific subject; or it might even provide online access to an entire professional publication, complete with text, pictures, letters to the editor, and advertisements. These server "sites" are accessed using a personal computer or a terminal that has appropriate client software—that is, software that understands the communication protocols being used by the server (Tomaiuolo, 1995). Z39.50 is a new "applications-layer protocol originally modeled within the Open Systems Interconnection (OSI) Basic Reference Model developed by the International Organization for Standardization" (Moen, 1992). It standardizes the way clients and servers communicate, "even when there are differences between computer systems, search engines, and databases," providing a sort of universal translator for electronic information exchange (Moen, 1992). This application opens new opportunities for information sharing among resident computer systems by eliminating some of the traditional client/server limitations. The only way to really appreciate the full capabilities of the Internet is to see and use it; to do so, contact other health sciences, academic, or public libraries, many of which have at least one publicly accessible Internet workstation where you can see how the different systems work.

The World Wide Web (the Web) is "the most recent, popular, and expanding facet of the Internet" (Raw & White, 1996, p. 286). The communication protocol for the Web is HyperText Transfer Protocol (HTTP); it enables text, audio, and images to be combined in one document. Using HyperText Markup Language (HTML), it links to separate documents or to information in different formats. HTML is a specific application of Standard Generalized Markup Language (SGML), "an international standard for the definition of device-independent, system-independent methods of representing texts in electronic form" (Boutell, 1996). These standardized formatting codes are fostered by the International Organization for Standardization (ISO). Browsers provide user interfaces that make navigating the Web relatively easy. Powerful search engines on the browsers allow the user to ask to see "sites" containing material related to a search statement. Then the user can "click" on highlighted parts of the screen to go to a "page" or "link" related to the requested information, which contain additional links.

Nursing associations and professionals are just beginning to explore the variety and complexity of research and practice opportunities the Web has to offer. Some sites require registration or membership to use specific services, such as access to specialized databases. Libraries that do not want to bother with the installation of CD-ROM databases may subscribe to major systems via the Web. Recently, major nursing publications have been made available on the World Wide Web, and subscriptions to these "electronic" journals are also available.

Librarians must consider exactly what benefits and risks are involved in switching to Web access, particularly in the area of electronic journals. For-fee online access to materials or systems usually requires a license that must be renewed periodically. Depending upon the license agreement regarding archival rights, electronic information may or may not be downloaded or printed in order to have an archival copy in the event that a subscription is cancelled. On the other hand, professional organizations that have determined print publication of new research is too costly may now be able to publish electronically at extremely low costs, thereby reducing, or even eliminating, charges for access. Further, there are many free Web sites of high quality, especially image banks in pathology or ultrasound, that are useful additions to the library's resources. These are usually maintained by professional organizations or associations, and are highly credible, although there is no guarantee that they will always be available on an as-needed basis. So much material is available on the Web that selecting useful sites can be a daunting and time-consuming task. This, however, is where the librarian can play an important role: locating, evaluating, and publicizing credible and useful uniform resource locators (URLs), the "addresses" of Web sites; and providing information on how to reference these sources.

In order to keep up with these opportunities, nursing libraries must provide users with access to the Web. Most academic institutions and a growing number of hospitals have Internet access. Commercial companies also vend Internet access. And thanks to recent legislation, telephone companies are now able to sell Internet access to customers. The library should contact a commercial vendor if no Internet access is provided through the parent institution.

Once the decision has been made to provide Internet access, the library will need to purchase computer hardware and software to support these services. This field of information science is changing rapidly, and specific packages for accessing and searching the Web are appearing almost daily. Professional journals in nursing, information science, and in the computing field are a good place to begin research, as myriad articles describe and evaluate various hardware and software configurations. Fortunately, once one has access to the Web, search engines can be used to locate online sites to keep up to date. Deciding which hardware to purchase also depends on the types of access the library intends to provide. A general rule is that one can never have too much disk space, especially when dealing with graphics, and one can never have too much memory (RAM), which affects the speed of retrieval. In addition, include laser printers as part of the equipment requirements, as they will be necessary to produce high-quality printouts of Web materials, and are particularly important if you must deal with color graphics. (Dot-matrix printers are "blind" to colors—that is, cannot print them.)

Last (and perhaps this should be considered first), when considering the purchase of any computer equipment, factor in the costs of either an uninterruptable power supply, or at the very least, a quality surge protector. Even in small libraries, it is probably advisable to purchase a tape backup machine. In large libraries, routine system backups should be done daily on systems (such as the catalog) that are used heavily, and at least monthly on other stations. And every personal workstation should have a set of "doomsday" disks that will reboot the system in an emergency. Finally, post vendor support phone numbers where they are easy to reference (do *not* put them in a computer file). The primary causes of computer failure are heat, dust, and power failures; therefore, set up workstations away from high-volume printers, and provide a separate air-conditioned room for large systems. Train staff to back up their files, and to maintenance their hard drives by routinely deleting data that is no longer relevant. And be sure to load virus-check programs on all systems that interface with networks, or on which users work with floppy disks. Most computer problems can be prevented with appropriate protection and routine maintenance.

COPYRIGHT, INTELLECTUAL FREEDOM, AND CONFIDENTIALITY

Copyright Legislation Regarding Print, Nonprint, and Digitized Information

Probably no other area of librarianship can spark long, heated, and emotional discussions as that of copyright; specifically, Federal Law (title 17, U.S. Code). (Note: The information here is not intended to serve as legal advice, permission, or direction. When confronted with issues of copyright, it is always best to consult a qualified attorney.) Although legal language can be confusing to non-attorneys, librarians nevertheless should read the section of the U.S. Code on copyright. Copyright is a form of protection provided by the laws of the United States to the authors of "original works of authorship" including literary, dramatic, musical, artistic, and certain other intellectual works. This protection is available to both published and unpublished works, and provides exclusive—but limited— rights to the owner of the copyright.

Fair Use. Sections 107 through 119 of the Copyright Act establish limitations on copyright protection; in some cases, in the form of specified exemptions from copyright liability. One major limitation is the doctrine of "fair use," which is given a statutory basis in section 107 of the act, and reproduced here.

Section 107. Limitations on exclusive rights: Fair use.

Notwithstanding the provisions of section 106 and 106A, the fair use of a copyrighted work, including such use by reproduction in copies of phonorecords or by any other means specified by that section, for purposes such as criticism, comment, news reporting, teaching (including multiple copies for

46

classroom use), scholarship, or research, is not an infringement of copyright.

In determining whether the use made of a work in any particular case is a fair use the factors to be considered shall include—

(1) the purpose and character of the use, including whether such use is of a commercial nature or is for nonprofit educational purposes;

(2) the nature of the copyrighted work;

(3) the amount and substantiality of the portion used in relation to the copyrighted work as a whole; and

(4) the effect of the use upon the potential market for or value of the copyrighted work.

The fact that a work is unpublished shall not itself bar a finding of fair use if such finding is made upon consideration of all the above factors.

This statement offers some guidance to users in determining when the principles of the doctrine apply, but the endless variety of situations and combinations of circumstances that can arise preclude the formulation of exact rules in the statute. In short, it is up to the courts to adapt the doctrine to particular situations on a case-by-case basis.

Section 108 of title 17, U.S. Code concerns "Reproduction by Libraries and Archives," which applies to library photocopying. Nothing contained in section 108 in any way affects the right of fair use—that is, no provision of section 108 is intended to remove any rights existing under the fair use doctrine. To the contrary, section 108 authorizes certain photocopying practices that may not qualify as fair use. The criteria of fair use are necessarily set forth in general terms, because in applying it to specific photocopying practices of libraries, an appropriate balancing of the rights of creators and the needs of users comes into play.

A wise recommendation in this regard is presented in section 108, clause (1), subsection (f), which states "That such [reproducing] equipment displays a notice that the making of a copy may be subject to the copyright law." This practice will be elaborated upon in the next section. For now, note that aside from being a provision of the law, a notice of this type will help to sensitize patrons to the issue and encourage them to exercise due diligence.

Section 108 also addresses interlibrary loan. The library or archive has privileges that do not exist for other establishments. Section 108 recognizes the services provided by libraries in the collection and distribution of information. Because interlibrary loan is an area where technologies are developing and expanding, the guidelines of the act provide guidance, not definitive answers. Awareness of these principles will assist in making decisions and arrangements for sharing the collection locally or globally.

Copyright Policies. Policies approved and implemented by institutional authority and adhered to by staff and patrons alike are instrumental in meeting the complex responsibilities itemized under the Copyright Act. "A policy establishes the institution's determination to adhere to copyright law, clarifies responsibility for infringements, communicates the need for observance of the law, and creates implementation and enforcement measures" (Vlcek, 1992, p. vii).

The purpose of a copyright policy is to spell out the provisions of the Copyright Act regarding the particular situation and issues of concern to the institution. Often there is little awareness or understanding of the law and difficulty interpreting its use. An established policy creates awareness of the need to comply, and can be used as a guide for directing individuals to appropriate persons or departments to find answers to questions regarding compliance. Librarians, information specialists, and archivists should be familiar with the basic principles to evaluate common concerns. For more complex issues or situations, legal advice is in order.

Finally, an institutional copyright policy, explaining what can and cannot be reproduced, can provide the foundation for the design of standardized forms used to obtain permissions. An individual can be designated to work with the librarian to follow through in the processing of the forms; or the librarian can engage the Copyright Clearance Center to facilitate the processing of copyright permissions.

For additional information on copyright law, access the LC Web site at http://lcweb.loc.gov/copyright/.

Intellectual Freedom and the ALA's Library Bill of Rights

In the late nineteenth century, in response to a growing number of threats to free and open access to library materials, the American Library Association (ALA) began to discuss and formulate what has since evolved into its present stand on intellectual freedom and the accompanying Library Bill of Rights (see Figure 2.1). Intellectual freedom as defined by the American Library Association encompasses a concept based on individuals' "right to hold any belief on any subject," to "convey their ideas in any form" and to have "unrestricted access to information and ideas . . . ." (Office for Intellectual Freedom, American Library Association, 1996, p. xiii). These ideas have evolved and changed over time, and certainly reflect the shifts in societal norms. Most librarians and laypeople consider public libraries as being in the position of having to defend these ideas. Who can forget the image of Bette Davis as the librarian/heroine in the movie *Storm Center*, fighting for the right to keep a book on communism on the shelves after a public outcry demanding its (and her) removal? In a somewhat less dramatic way, these principles apply to academic and corporate libraries, although the ways these ideas are put forth and protected may vary according to institutional values and standards.

No matter what the type of institutional setting, the library usually endeavors to be the "Switzerland" of information resources, providing access to a variety of published opinions and research on whatever subject area is being supported, without bias toward any particular set of beliefs. The same should hold true for a nursing information center. Although nursing materials on the surface would not seem to be cause for conflict, unexpected situations can develop into full-blown controversies if not handled properly. The following are some possible scenarios:

- A nursing faculty member in a church-affiliated college of nursing or hospital library demands that all books be removed on counseling patients after abortion.

The Library Bill of Rights

The American Library Association affirms that all libraries are forums for information and ideas, and that the following basic policies should guide their services.

I. Books and other library resources should be provided for the interest information, and enlightenment of all people of the community the library serves. Materials should not be excluded because of the origin, background, or views of those contributing to their creation.

II. Libraries should provide materials and information presenting all points of view on current and historical issues. Materials should not be proscribed or removed because of partisan or doctrinal disapproval.

III. Libraries should challenge censorship in the fulfillment of their responsibility to provide information and enlightenment.

IV. Libraries should cooperate with all persons and groups concerned with resisting abridgment of free expression and free access to ideas.

V. A person's right to use a library should not be denied or abridged because of origin, age, background, or views.

VI. Libraries which make exhibit spaces and meeting rooms available to the public they serve should make such facilities on an equitable basis, regardless of the beliefs of affiliations of individuals or groups requesting their use.

Adopted June 18, 1948. Amended by the ALA Council February 2, 1961; June 27, 1967; and January 23, 1980. (Office for Intellectual Freedom, American Library Association, 1996, pp. 3–4).
Reprinted with the permission of the American Library Association.

Figure 2.1   The Library Bill of Rights

- A physician in a traditional (Western) medical setting objects to books in the collection on alternative treatments and therapies, referring to them as "quackery."
- A physician requests that information not be provided to a certain patient because "he or she is not ready to hear it yet."
- A nurse asks for information to use in forming a union within the hospital.

Collection Development Policies. Patient care settings, particularly those in an educational program, reflect many issues of concern to society in general. Ideally, a library's collection development policy will address in great detail the subject areas targeted for the collection (see Chapter 5 for additional information). The collection development policy, which should be approved by the institution's library committee or other advisory body, is the basic guideline and standard for all materials being added to the collection. For some individuals and institutions, materials that represent new, unusual, or unpopular ideas are threatening, and their first reaction may be to attempt to remove them. The best advice is to anticipate those items that might cause controversy and be ready with the rationale for their inclusion.

In addition, clients (nursing personnel as well as students) will request bibliographic searches or interlibrary loan materials that encompass controversial topics. For example, one librarian who provided information on union organizing to a member of the nursing staff was later reprimanded by upper-level hospital administration for doing so. Another librarian helped someone from outside the institution find information on one of the trustees and was told in no uncertain terms that such information was considered confidential by the administrators of her institution. These examples point out that, in the corporate setting of the hospital, what is good for the client might not always be good for the parent (or supporting) institution. Thus, it is important that policies for retrieving (or not retrieving) these materials be clearly defined, and that the library committee support those policies. It is also important to ascertain that no individual librarian's personal biases interfere with his or her willingness to fill requests for information.

Right to Privacy. Another area addressed by the Library Bill of Rights concerns a client's right to privacy in his or her use of library materials. Challenges to this generally come from someone in the parent organization (for example, a faculty member or hospital administrator) seeking information about a student's or employee's reading habits or requests for information. A more innocent scenario is when one employee or student wants to know who has checked out a book so that he or she might contact that person in order to use it. Regardless, the client's right to privacy should be protected in all cases, otherwise the concept of "free and open access" is compromised.

Often there is an easy way to safeguard individual privacy while accommodating a request. In the case of an unavailable book, one common solution is to have the librarian or staff member call the client who has the item. In an institution where original research is taking place and faculty and researchers are competing for grant monies, it is even more important to respect the privacy of individual clients. In a clinical patient setting, confidentiality is mandated, which certainly extends to patients in the library requesting information and background on their medical conditions. It is essential to instruct volunteers, student workers, and any other staff in these basic tenets of the Library Bill of Rights to ensure that they are carried out consistently.

The American Library Association's *Intellectual Freedom Manual* (Office for Intellectual Freedom, 1996) explains these issues in great detail, and should be referenced by anyone forming policies for a new library.

STANDARDS, EVALUATION, AND ACCREDITATION

Library Standards

The area of standards can be confusing even to the experienced librarian, because there is no one authoritative body to which all libraries can look for these standards. For example, the American Library Association, the Association for College & Research Libraries, the Special Libraries Association, and the Medical Library

Association all publish standards that might apply and be useful to a nursing library or information center.

The purpose of standards is to provide a baseline set of criteria for library operations, and they should be considered during the planning phase. On a political level, published standards make a good selling point with a library committee or board. Being able to point to something "official" such as a published set of standards may make it easier to obtain committee approval or funding for some basic level of service such as interlibrary loan. The published standards of the Association of College & Research Libraries ("Standards for College Libraries," 1986), address library objectives, collections, organization of materials, staff, services, facilities, administration, and budgets.

Evaluation of Programs and Services

Libraries often neglect to engage in any ongoing evaluation of programs and services, even though this is an area that is becoming more essential as budgets continue to shrink and demands for accountability continue to grow. The point of organizing and offering library services is to support the information needs of a particular clientele whether it is nursing staff within a hospital, an undergraduate baccalaureate student group, or the faculty who teach in a nursing education setting. Without some form of evaluation, it will be impossible to determine whether the clientele is getting the informational support they need.

Evaluation processes make it possible to objectively determine whether a service is effective or should be changed or streamlined. Data generated from measuring services can make the difference between a successful and unsuccessful plea for more staffing. For the library, carefully kept statistics demonstrate the use of the collection, staff time management, budget needs, guides for deselection, areas of improvement, and viability—to name a few. Contracts and receipts from business transactions provide records as proof of activity.

Statistics are a means of painting a picture of activities that directly relate to the mission and goals of the library. Statistical reports, whether daily, weekly, or monthly, provide an important means for evaluating and reevaluating how best to use available resources. For example, statistics kept on interlibrary loan materials can, after a period of time, indicate the need to purchase particular journals or titles. These same interlibrary loan statistics can indicate the strengths of the collection when combined with regular circulation figures.

There are many different methods and levels of evaluating library services and processes, ranging from broad user-satisfaction surveys to studying the turnaround time of interlibrary loan requests (Van House, Weil, & McClure, 1990, p. 5). Evaluation is simply another step in the planning process, and the results from such studies can keep the planning process alive by providing invaluable feedback and ideas for growth and change. Even in a small library, it is possible to collect valuable data without much difficulty. At the very least, it is advisable to monthly keep statistics on "how much" the library provides in each service; for example, how many interlibrary loans and literature searches were requested and filled, or the number of items circulated. These types of numbers imply work accomplished, and charted over time, might be a clear indicator of the need for more personnel.

Sometimes, it is possible to collect a number of different data elements about a service at once. For instance, if the mediated literature search service were being studied, data could be collected on:

- Turnaround time (the length of time measured from receipt of the request to delivering the material to the client).
- Type of client requesting the search (student, clinician, or faculty, etc.).
- Databases searched.
- Degree to which the client was satisfied with the end product (with subcategories for more specific questions reflecting the client's opinion of the relevance of the search results).

The data collected for each of the points just listed may provide some valuable feedback for improving the service, or validate a librarian's perception that a particular service is working well. Or such data may reveal that turnaround time is significantly longer than suspected, which would lead to an evaluation of the entire process to make it more efficient, showing, perhaps, that requests could be filled faster if the library used fax machines or the Internet for transmitting documents instead of the U.S. mail.

It is also essential to study who in the client population is requesting a service, to determine whether the target group is being served. The fact, for example, that no registered nurses in the hospital are requesting literature searches from the library may indicate that more marketing of the service should be aimed toward this group to heighten their awareness of the service.

Likewise, examining which databases the librarians are searching may determine whether they are taking full advantage of the range of databases available. It not uncommon for librarians to fall into a rut of searching only those databases with which they are most familiar.

Finally, it is necessary to learn whether the results are actually helpful to the client in order to determine whether the original goal of providing the service is being met. If clients do not consistently rate the results of the literature searches as relevant, this could point to a need for more training in conducting the searches. Or it may be that the interviewing process should be reviewed to make sure that the proper questions are being asked of the client before the search is carried out. Commonly, a client will ask a reference question in the beginning of an interview that is somewhat removed from the actual need. This situation extends to requests for literature searches as well.

Data collection, it should be noted, need not always involve the client directly. In the preceding example, all the data except for client satisfaction could be gleaned from the search request form itself—which is not to say that direct client feedback is not extremely valuable. If the overall goal of the library is to serve the client's needs, nothing carries quite as much weight as the client's opinion of the effectiveness of those services.

When planning evaluation studies of library services, it is important to tie the study as closely as possible to the long-term planning goals and objectives of the library. Other areas of study might be found by examining the various accreditation criteria that the library will have to address when the institution comes up for formal accreditation.

Although it may be necessary to maintain ongoing statistics on some services to track staffing needs, it probably is not necessary to conduct evaluations on all services at all times. A better idea is to focus on a particular service to study closely, looking for methods of improvement, and subsequently implementing any needed changes, followed by another study after the change has had time to make an impact. It is also easier to maintain a higher level of staff interest and enthusiasm for participating in evaluation if there is a beginning and end point to each study.

Accreditation

Accreditation is a voluntary process whereby a program or institution undergoes an extensive review and evaluation according to standards or criteria published by the accrediting body. Essentially, an institution must provide proof that it has accomplished what it claimed it would. Because accreditation can be both time-consuming and costly, and is technically voluntary, why do institutions put themselves through this process? In short, it would be very difficult for an institution to survive without it. Local, state, and federal funding (at the very least, student financial aid) is often tied to an institution's accreditation (Williams, 1993, p. 32). Even more important than funding perhaps is the institution's reputation. Often, job prerequisites include a degree from an accredited institution, therefore, a prospective student may choose not to participate in an unaccredited program when other accredited programs are available.

A less-tangible reward is that the accreditation process by its very nature puts the institution into a planning and evaluation mode, and helps pave the way for change. It is all too easy to fall into a routine that precludes change. Finally, accreditation is an affirmation from a peer group that the institution or program is of merit.

Currently there are three types of accreditation:

1. *Institutional.* A review of the educational institution as a whole with an overall look at all of its programs and services. Currently, there are six regional accrediting bodies that carry out accreditation of educational institutions (Sacks & Whildin, 1993):

   Middle States Association of Colleges and Schools

   New England Association of Schools and Colleges

   North Central Association of Colleges and Schools

   Northwest Association of Schools and Colleges

   Southern Association of Colleges and Schools

   Western Association of Schools and Colleges

2. *Program/specialized/professional.* This type of accreditation is program-specific rather than institutionwide, and the accreditation body is usually the recognized accrediting body within that profession. Currently, the National League for Nursing (NLN) accredits degree, diploma, and practical nursing programs

3. *State agency.* Professional programs often carry the additional requirement that they be approved or accredited by a state agency. In the case of a nursing program, it is the state board of nursing that handles this accreditation.

Program and state agency accreditation (or approval) often begins with a prerequisite of regional accreditation (so much for the voluntary nature of accreditation). In the case of a diploma nursing program based in a hospital, the prerequisite accreditation would be that the hospital itself is accredited by the Joint Commission on Accreditation of Healthcare Organizations (JCAHO).

An example of a possible accreditation scenario might be the following: Northwest College, a four-year liberal arts college in Oregon, offers a Bachelor of Science in Nursing. To be considered "fully" accredited, the college as a whole must first pass regional accreditation with the Northwest Association of Schools and Colleges. The School of Nursing would have to undergo examination and receive approval by the Oregon State Board of Nursing; finally, the program would have to be accredited by the NLN.

The focus of this discussion is NLN accreditation since it is common to all nursing programs whether baccalaureate, diploma, or master's or higher-degree programs. The NLN Board of Governors, which is accountable to the Council on Post-secondary Accreditation (COPA) and to the U.S. Department of Education, is ultimately responsible for the accreditation of nursing programs (National League for Nursing, 1990, p. 4). There are six steps or stages in NLN accreditation (National League for Nursing, 1990, p. 7):

1. *Determination of eligibility for initial evaluation.* An institution must pass certain requirements before it can even request accreditation by the NLN. One of these requirements is that other state and regional accreditation must already be in place before the NLN will begin the process of accreditation.

2. *Initiation of the process.* For first-time accreditation, once an institution has determined (with help from the NLN) that it is truly ready to undergo the process, the chief officer of the parent institution formally applies for accreditation with the NLN. Programs that are already accredited will be notified when the time for renewal is approaching.

3. *Self-study process and writing the self-study report.* Criteria and guidelines issued by the NLN (or other accrediting agency) will be addressed systematically in the self-study report. Essentially, the report will examine and self-evaluate every aspect of the program and its role within the larger institution. The NLN has one criterion that specifically addresses library services in all three of its program criteria. Additionally, there are pertinent factors pertaining to the library under the physical facilities criteria.

4. *The accreditation visit.* The accreditation visit itself is conducted by nurses in the field who have been specially trained for this step. The visit usually occurs over the course of three to five days, and involves several site visitors, who systematically tour and observe various parts of the program in action. The library is usually included in this tour and the visitors may want to schedule time with the librarian. Since no one will be able to better demonstrate the effectiveness of the library's participation in institutional and program goals, the librarian or manager of the library should actively campaign to present personally this aspect of the self-study. The findings of the team are presented at the end of the visit, and basically serve to verify facts and materials presented in the self-study. They include the team's recommendation as to whether the program should be granted full, partial, or no accreditation.

5. *Evaluation.* Evaluation here refers to the final review of the program applying for accreditation. Although the site visitors represent the accrediting body and make a recommendation, the final authority rests with the appropriate board of review within the NLN that has been made responsible for granting accreditation. Most of the time, the board accepts the recommendation of the visiting team, but there have been cases where the board has not. Thus, the granting of accreditation is not final until the board issues its decision.

6. *Systematic program of ongoing evaluation.* Once accreditation has been awarded, a nursing program is expected to carry out an ongoing process of examination and evaluation that will serve as the basis for the next self-study report and bid for accreditation renewal. Feedback from the site visitors should be incorporated into subsequent self-study reports.

In total, the formal process of accreditation can last several years from beginning to end, but in fact never really ends because those involved in administering a program are always reviewing and evaluating the program in preparation for the next accreditation period.

The role of the librarian in the accreditation process will vary according to the institution and type of accreditation, but will be particularly important in any educational program. A library's role in accreditation, although only one part of the overall picture, will nonetheless be an important one since it serves the entire institution. Early in the planning stages for accreditation, the librarian should petition to be appointed to committees being formed and to be active in the entire process ("Tips for librarians planning for accreditation visits," 1992). Certainly, if the accreditation concerns a nursing program, it would be advisable for the librarian to participate in any general meetings of the nursing faculty working on the self-study. This will result not only in being better prepared for the site visit but will undoubtedly result in better planning and evaluation for the future. A thorough knowledge and understanding of the criteria and guidelines of the accrediting agency are essential to the process. The institutional liaison should provide everyone involved in the process with a copy of these criteria.

During the process of accreditation, the institution may consider employing consultants to serve as advisors in guiding the institution through the accreditation process—answering questions that arise and clarifying points of confusion. The librarian should take advantage of this opportunity and query the consultants on any current trends that may be taking place in how the accreditation teams look at library facilities and services. With the Internet and current technology making it easy to communicate with peers across the country, e-mail and listservs are another amazingly easy and global method of getting feedback from others who have recently been through the process. There are various nursing and library listserv discussion groups where such questions would be appropriate. This is an excellent no-cost method for getting more detailed advice and suggestions about the site visit from others who have successfully completed the accreditation process.

CONCLUSION

Some of the basic elements for planning and developing a library or information center have been addressed in this chapter. Succeeding chapters and additional readings will present information on issues pertinent to specific library functions. It is important to understand the overall organizational structure and management of nursing information in order to set the context for further refinement in individual cases. The mission statement frames many policies and procedures, laying the groundwork for the support of professional needs by continuous improvement in the quality of access and services. External evaluation, accreditation processes, and internal performance review, integrate a system of information management directed toward serving the data and knowledge expectations to support nursing education, practice, and administration.

REFERENCES

Boutell, T. (1996). World Wide Web FAQ. [On-Online]. Available: http://gamma.is.tcu.edu/~taylor/htmfaq/index.htm.

Cibbarelli, P. R., Gertel, E. H., & Kratzert, M. (1993). Choosing among the options for patron access databases. Print, online, CD-ROM, or locally mounted. Reference Librarian, 39, 85–97.

Darling, L., Bishop, D., & Colaianni, L. A. (Eds.). (1982). Handbook of medical library practice: Vol. 3. Health science librarianship and administration. Chicago: Medical Library Association.

Directory of the Medical Library Association, Medical Library Association 1995/96. (1995). Chicago: Medical Library Association.

Ka-Neg, A. (1992). Hardware options: From LANs to WANs. CD-ROM Librarian, 7(3), 12–17.

Mates, B. (1992). Adaptive technology makes libraries "people friendly." Computers in Libraries, 12(10), 20–24.

Michaels, A., & Michaels, D. (1992). Designing for technology in today's libraries. Computers in Libraries, 12(1), 8–15.

Moen, W. (1992). The ANSI/NISO Z39.50 protocol: Informational retrieval in the information infrastructure. [On-line]. Available: http://www.cni.org/pub/NISO/docs/Z39.50-1992/www/50.brochure.toc.html.

Moore, J. A., & Vincent, J. A. (1994). Strategic and tactical planning: From corporate level to department Level. In J. J. Hampton (Ed.), AMA *management handbook* (3rd ed., pp. 1–36). New York: American Management Association.

National League for Nursing. (1990). *Policies and procedures of accreditation for programs in nursing education.* New York: Author.

Office for Intellectual Freedom, American Library Association. (1996). *Intellectual freedom manual.* Chicago: American Library Association.

Raw, A., & White, K. (1996). Nurses' guide to the Internet—AORN online. *AORN Journal, 64,* 286, 289.

Sacks, P. A., & Whildin, S. L. (1993). *Preparing for accreditation.* Chicago: American Library Association.

Schockley, J. S. (1988). *Information sources for nursing, a guide.* New York: National League for Nursing.

Standards for college libraries, 1986. (1986). *College and Research Library News, 3,* 189–200.

Tips for librarians planning for accreditation visits. (1992). *College and Research Library News, 7,* 447.

Tomaiuolo, N. G. (1995). Accessing nursing resources on the Internet. *Computers in Nursing, 13,* 159–164.

Van House, N. A., Weil, B. T., & McClure, C. R. (1990). *Measuring academic library performance: A practical approach.* Chicago: American Library Association.

Vlcek, C. W. (1992). *Adoptable copyright policy and manual designed for adoption by schools, colleges & universities.* Washington, DC: Copyright Information Services.

Wilkinson, D. (1992). Multiple database operation on the stand-alone public CD-ROM system: Considerations for system management. *CD-ROM Librarian, 7*(7), 22–28.

Williams, D. E. (1993). Accreditation and the academic library. *Library Administration and Management, 7,* 31–37.

RESOURCE REFERENCES

Blair, M. K., Williams, M. A., Rand, P. S., & Schanno, M. T. (1994). Building the library/information center of the future: A resource guide. *Computer Methods and Programs in Biomedicine, 44,* 263–266.

Bradley, J. (Ed.). (1983). *Hospital library management.* Chicago: Medical Library Association. (Dated, but some of the information is still valid.)

Bridges, A., & Thede, L. Q. (1996). Electronic education: Nursing education resources on the World Wide Web. *Nurse Educator, 21*(5), 11–15.

Bruwelheide, J. H. (1995). *The copyright primer for librarians and educators* (3rd ed.). Chicago: American Library Association.

Christianson, E. B., King, D. E., & Ahrensfeld, J. L. (1991). *Special libraries: A guide for management*. Chicago: Special Libraries Association.

Cibbarelli, P. (1996). Library automation alternatives in 1996 and user satisfaction ratings of library users by operating system. *Computers in Libraries, 16*(2), 26–35.

Copyright Information Services. (1992). *Official fair use guidelines* (4th ed.). Washington, DC: Author.

Czepiel, J. A., Solomon, M. R., & Surprenant, C. F. (1985). *The service encounter: Managing employee/customer interaction in a service business*. Lexington, MA: Lexington Books.

Gonzalez, E. L. F., & Seaton, H. J. (1995). Internet sources for nursing and allied health. *Database, 18*, 46–49.

Medical Library Association, Task Force on the Role of the Librarian. (1996). *Step one: MLA's librarian survival kit*. Chicago: Medical Library Association.

National League for Nursing. (1990). *Policies and procedures of accreditation for programs in nursing education* (6th ed.). New York: Author.

National League for Nursing, Council of Baccalaureate and Higher Degree Programs. (1991). *Criteria and guidelines for the evaluation of baccalaureate and higher degree programs in nursing*. New York: National League for Nursing.

National League for Nursing, Council of Diploma Programs. (1991). *Criteria and guidelines for the evaluation of diploma programs in nursing*. New York: National League for Nursing.

National League for Nursing, Council of Practical Nursing Programs. (1991). *Criteria and guidelines for the evaluation of practical nursing programs*. New York: National League for Nursing.

Office for Intellectual Freedom, American Library Association. (1996). *Intellectual freedom manual*. Chicago: American Library Association.

Perone, K. (1996). Networking CD-ROMs: A tutorial introduction. *Computers in Libraries, 16*(2), 71–77.

Sacks, P. A., & Whildin, S. L. (1993). *Preparing for accreditation*. Chicago: American Library Association.

Sager, D. J. (1992). *Small libraries: Organization and operation*. Fort Atkinson, WI: Highsmith Press.

St. Clair, G., & Williamson, J. (1992). *Managing the new one-person library*. London: Bowker Saur.

Standards Committee, Hospital Libraries Section, Medical Library Association. (1994). *Standards for hospital libraries*. Chicago: Medical Library Association.

Vlcek, C. W. (1992). *Adoptable copyright policy and manual designed for adoption by schools, colleges & universities*. Washington, DC: Copyright Information Services.

Young, K. E., Chambers, C. M., Kells, H. R., & Associates. (1983). *Understanding accreditation*. San Francisco: Jossey-Bass.

SUGGESTED READINGS

Ayre, R. (1994). Making the Internet connection. *PC Magazine, 13*(17), 118–122, 126, 128, 132, 134–135.

Ives, D. J. (1996). Security management strategies for protecting your library's network. *Computers in Libraries, 16*(2), 36–41.

Jarred, A. D., & Coleman, P. (1994). Regional association criteria and the Standards for College Libraries: The informal role of quantitative input measures for libraries in accreditation. *The Journal of Academic Librarianship, 20*, 273–284.

Kara, B., Caputo, A., & Davis, T. (1995). Negotiating contracts for electronic resources. *The Serials Librarian, 25*, 269–275.

Marousky, R. T. (1996). Nurses' guide to the Internet—Purchasing a home computer system and getting connected. *AORN Journal, 64*, 112–114.

McCarthy, C. A. (1996). Volunteers and technology: The new reality. *American Libraries, 27*, 67–73.

Mosley, S., Caggiano, A., & Charles, J. (1996). The "Self-Weeding" collection: The ongoing problem of library theft, and how to fight back. *Library Journal, 121*(17), 38–40.

Prohaska, J. L., & Chang, B. L. (1996). Computer use and nursing research: Using the Internet to enhance nursing knowledge and practice. *Western Journal of Nursing Research, 18*, 365–370.

Sellen, M. (1991). Specialized accreditation and the library. *Collection Building, 11*(3), 2–8.

Witt, T. B. (1996). The use of electronic book theft detection systems in libraries. *Journal of Interlibrary Loan, Document Delivery & Information Supply, 6*(4), 45–60.

3

Basic Considerations in Administration: Budgeting, Personnel Management, and Public Relations

Dawn Bick, BNSc, MLS, AHIP
Deborah L. Graham, MLS

The purpose of this chapter is to take some of the mystery out of financial planning and related activities. It views finance as the broad process of managing money and other assets, and focuses on budgeting as a means of developing a systematic plan for generating revenue and meeting expenses within a specified time period. Grants and fund-raising, important extensions of budgetary activity, are also discussed, along with the administrative areas of personnel management and public relations.

THE LIBRARY BUDGET AND THE INSTITUTIONAL BUDGET

The concepts of finance and budget continue to cause anxiety to those charged with administering a library, often because many first-time managers assume their responsibilities with little or no experience in formulating a budget document, much less dealing with the politics of the budgeting process. Often, a basic understanding of accounting principles is lacking. Even experienced library managers find that their expertise in the area of finance falls short of what particular situations require.

A nursing library may be organized in a number of ways. It may be a specialized operation serving an association, corporate body, or nursing program; it may be a hospital or academic department or part of a larger such department; it may be integrated within a larger hospital or health sciences library; or it may be integrated within a general academic library. But no matter what the setting, the process of financing the library and its operations follows similar steps.

Black (1993) points out that the process of budgeting places the library's strategic plan into a financial framework, wherein the budget reflects the library's goals and objectives by directing resources to priority services, programs, and so on. As such, the budget can also be an effective measure of the library's accomplishments and performance. When the budget is tied to the library's plan in this way, it becomes a dynamic managerial tool as opposed to a static accounting system. Budgets can become our friends!

Stoffle (1992) details three major stages in the budget process: development and securement, allocation, and management. She describes the importance of each stage and indicates the necessity for understanding the major players involved and the effects of various tactical approaches. In the development phase, for example, it is critical to understand how the library fits in to the parent institution's budget situation, whether it be a hospital, association, college, or university. It is also essential that the library's goals be consistent with those of the institution and be communicated in that way. Consulting with a wide base of individuals including library staff and clients, business personnel, and interested parties from other departments results in support that may manifest itself in a number of ways down the line. "Crying poor" to these people will not work, however; all units in any given institution are being asked to do more with less, and the library is no exception. Rather, the approach by the library manager is to educate potential supporters on how the services and programs proposed by the library will further the goals of the institution in a cost-effective manner, and that the library is a sound investment. This education is an ongoing process and should take place on a daily basis, not just at budget time.

Phillip King, comptroller at the Houston Academy of Medicine–Texas Medical Center Library, recommends that any budget proposal be thoroughly reviewed by an accounting professional. This individual would ensure that there are no mathematical errors, that supporting schedules tie into summary pages, that costs seem reasonable with current costs, that planned activities are associated with related expenses, and that sufficient back-up information is available to answer questions that may arise during the allocation process.

When the actual written budget document is prepared, it has to be done so with the various supporters and audiences in mind. The format of the formal budget is usually prescribed by the parent institution, but other formats can and should be used to communicate the information to different parties for various purposes. For example, a hospital administrator may require only a short overview or an executive summary, whereas a division or department head is served best by more detail and comparisons to other budget years. The library staff needs to know how the budget figures affect particular services and how they can make the budget work best for them.

Once the proposed budget has been presented to institutional administration, the allocation process begins. Rarely are budgets accepted as submitted; usually there are several revisions before final approval. External allocation by the parent institution administration may earmark some budget lines, such as collections and personnel, but designate a lump sum for others to be decided internally. Again, it is recommended that there be broad involvement of staff in the internal allocations as long as it is clear who has the final word. Participation by those who will be implementing budget decisions will create a "buyin" to the final document and will contribute to more effective budget management.

Budget management throughout the year is a challenge to say the least. The foremost consideration is that progress toward the library's goals be monitored. In this way, use of funds can be "corrected" or even reallocated depending on current priorities. It is most desirable that the library manager have reallocation authority. If this is not possible, then an avenue for negotiating alternative uses of funds should be set up with the appropriate administrator at the outset of the budget cycle. Monitoring and spending the annual budget in a strategic and creative fashion and relating it to outcomes that support the institution's mission establishes a credibility that will be critical in successful negotiation of the next budget.

Budgeting Basics

Operating and Capital Expenditures. No matter which type of budget the library manager is called upon to prepare, it is critical to distinguish between operating and capital expenditures. Operating expenditures are those of a recurring nature, which are required to conduct daily business; examples are salaries, benefits, rent, and supplies. Capital expenditures are generally one-time in nature, have a long lifetime of usefulness, or long period recurring; examples are office furniture, carpeting, and bookshelving. Ideally, the future replacement costs should be calculated and amortized over a designated period and credited to a capital replacement or reserve fund. The parent institution often has this responsibility, but in some cases the library retains it.

Financial and Managerial Accounting. Financial accounting refers to the bookkeeping methods involved in recording the financial transactions of a business, preparing budget-to-actual expense analysis, and preparing statements of assets and liabilities for external review. The parent institution will dictate the type of financial accounting that is practiced, but it is helpful to understand the types and reasons a particular one is being used. Stanley (1993) presents a clear description of organizational accounting systems. In the cash basis of accounting, expenses are recorded in the period in which the cash payment is made, and revenues are recorded when cash payment is received. In accrual accounting, expenses and revenues are recorded in the period in which they are incurred. The Financial Accounting Standards Board (FASB) recommends the accrual method of accounting for libraries and most nonprofit institutions. The accrual system has the advantage of emphasizing the effects of services rendered or consumed on the business, as it matches revenue with related expenses for a given period of time. Accrual accounting also allows end-of-year adjusting of entries so that related revenues and expenditures can be recorded in the same fiscal year.

Understanding and using the accrual system of accounting will prepare the library manager well for institutional audit activity. An audit is a review of the main components of an institution's financial systems, during which auditors use standard techniques including process-flow analysis, verification of procedures, validation of specific transactions, interviews with employees and clients, and risk analysis. Following the prescribed accounting method enables a "clean" audit opinion on the financial statements, a statement of the fairness of the financial statements. If financial statements are prepared on a basis other than what is prescribed, the auditors can offer only a "qualified opinion," which indicates that the audited information is misleading in some way.

Managerial accounting refers to the types of internal accounting reports that are used by managers, department heads, supervisors, and others to support decision making. These reports have no prescribed format or frequency and present very detailed financial data about specific services or programs. They provide a means for the manager to track changes and make cost control and organizational adjustments as necessary. For example, equipment purchase or leasing decisions can be made on the basis of a detailed managerial report, which would include maintenance costs and so on.

Special and Restricted Funds. The concept of a capital reserve fund was introduced in the section on operating and capital expenditures. Examples of other special funds are endowments, memorial book funds, and building funds. Accessing and expending monies from these funds usually require special conditions and permissions that are established when the funds are created.

Dawn Bick & Deborah Graham

Types of Budgets

Line-Item Budgets. Black (1993) describes the line-item budget as "primarily an accounting system that calls for a review of annual expenditures for the year and a projection of costs in broad categories (lines) for the following year." The budget lines are applied to the library as a whole such that all salaries appear in one line item, all benefits in another, and so forth. Figure 3.1 shows a traditional line-item budget format.

There is no magic formula that dictates a specific percentage of the budget that should be earmarked for personnel, collections, and administration. Wages and benefits for personnel usually account for the largest portion of a library's budget, with collections next, followed by administration/supplies/equipment. The library manager needs to direct budget monies to products, services, and technologies that meet the needs and priorities of the library's clientele. In a time of change in the health care system and increasing options for access to information, flexibility is a key ingredient here.

Acct. #	Acct. Name	FY Proposed Budget	Comments	Prev. FY Budget	Prev. FY Projected Expenditures
####	Salaries				
####	Benefits				
####	Books				
####	Journals				
####	Office supplies				
####	Capitalized furniture, equipment				

Figure 3.1 Traditional Line-Item Budget Format

70

The budget format in Figure 3.1 is very useful for institutional accounting purposes and to justify general tracking of expenditures. Indeed, this format may be an institutional requirement. However, the process of taking the previous fiscal year's expenditures and incrementing them to reflect inflation does little to convince an administrator that anything dynamic and useful is being accomplished by the library. Since institutions are not in a financial position to automatically increment budgets from various units and departments, a more convincing argument needs to be made for any proposed budget increases and/or reallocation of funds. The program-based type of budget enables such arguments and can be used internally even if line-item budgets are required by the institution.

Program-Based Budgets. Black (1993) and Robinson and Robinson (1994) describe in detail the concept of program-based budgeting. This type of budget relates expenditures to particular library programs, services, and products. Thus, funds can be allocated according to the relative importance of particular programs, and the budget becomes a financial reflection of the library's service priorities. This is not an easy task and requires the traditional line-item budget to be completely restructured. It further requires that the library define its programs and services and create a cost center budget for each, determine the full cost of operating the library by enhancing the line-item budget, and allocate each category of cost in the enhanced budget to one or more of the cost centers. Figure 3.2 shows one library service and its cost center categories.

In order to reflect the true cost of operating the library, the traditional line-item budget can be "enhanced" by identifying costs that ordinarily do not appear in it. For example, in-kind contributions such as the cost of the space that houses the library and is provided by the parent organization can be calculated. In addition, the annual cost of capital services can be determined. Robinson and Robinson detail how all these costs can be allocated to individual cost centers. The resulting program budget provides the library manager with the true costs of providing services, down to the unit level (e.g., the cost of answering a reference

Cost Center	Cost Category	FY Proposed Budget	Comments	Prev. FY Budget	Prev. FY Projected Expenditures
Collection management	Acquisitions				
	Cataloging				
	Physical processing & binding				
	Deselecting, weeding & withdrawal				
	Book repair				
	Preservation				
	Shelving				

Figure 3.2   Program-Based Budget Format

question) if desired. This type of information is enormously help-ful in making management decisions about the kinds of services the library should provide and how the library should be orga-nized and funded to provide them. With the increasing emphasis on outcome assessment, cost data can be used for cost-benefit analyses related to the parent institution's mission.

Budget Monitoring and Cost-Cutting Strategies

The importance of monitoring expenditures and making budget re-visions throughout the year has already been noted. The library manager must be vigilant in this task and must employ cost-cutting strategies whenever possible without jeopardizing the accomplish-ment of the library's goals. Nielsen (1992/1993) discusses 10 "quick and dirty" cost-cutting strategies that can provide guidance for limiting expenditures. These strategies include reexamining individual costs, reevaluating work and looking for efficiencies, recycling, providing training for employees to keep skills up to date, utilizing employees' talents to best advantage, negotiating with vendors for better rates, evaluating and streamlining the library's organization, engaging in projects that best suit the library, working with the staff to generate suggestions on how to save time, and being sensitive to opportunities to change.

Fund-Raising and Grants

The Fund-Raising Process. Burlingame (1994) states that ongoing fund-raising is a key to any library's future. The need to provide more services with less resources has prompted library managers to look beyond the funding provided by the parent organization or institution. Ideally, a library will have multiple sources of support, and it is incumbent upon the library manager to seek these out and maintain them. White (1992) cautions that outside funds should be raised for "extra and special services that normal budgets cannot be expected to cover." The institutional management structure should still be held accountable for funding libraries adequately enough to carry on their basic business.

A successful library development program depends on the ability of the library to clearly articulate its mission. From this mission, an assessment of the library's needs can be conducted, and particular needs can be targeted for external funding. Indeed, matching the library's needs with a potential donor's wishes is a key to successful fund-raising.

It is critical that the library manager determine institutional limits on the nature and extent of fund-raising allowed and that efforts be coordinated with other units, divisions, and departments. Larger institutions usually have a development office that coordinates such activities. In a smaller setting, direct communication with administration may be the way to proceed.

Lapsley (1995) lists a number of questions that determine a library's readiness to solicit external funding. Included are the following:

73

Can you demonstrate a valid, urgent need for the funds?

Can you show that your library is the one best suited to meet this need?

Is yours a realistic solution with a reasonable budget and timetable?

Can you measure the results?

Do you have a plan for continuing the project without on-going external support?

Can you show how the donor will benefit by making such a gift?

Sirota (1992) describes the fund-raising process in detail, noting that successful fund-raising "must be time-effective and cost-effective, and must seek to maintain interest in your institution and its needs." Six funding sources are identified as "individuals, businesses and corporations, foundations, government agencies, community-based service organizations, and owned endowments and investments." He goes on to list seven steps in fund-raising:

1. Develop a mission statement.
2. Research for possible donors.
3. Rate potential donors.
4. Cultivate donor prospects.
5. Solicit cash, goods, services, volunteers.
6. Acknowledge donor responses.
7. Sustain relationships by stewardship.

The importance of articulating the library's mission statement and relating proposed projects to it has already been discussed. Donor research is an unfamiliar area for many library managers, but it is an extremely important one. A systematic research plan will result in the best way to approach a specific donor. Tucker (1992) indicates that there are four kinds of information needed about potential donors: a biographical profile, an in-depth financial assessment, giving preferences, and the best solicitor (i.e., who is your best contact with this donor?). The format of information-gathering needs to be predetermined to ensure consistency and completeness; the depth of research including time limits, record maintenance, and staffing must be planned. Because most libraries do not have dedicated staff to perform these tasks, managers have to figure out a way to address them. Creative staffing and use of volunteers for routine clerical functions are promising options to enable even the smallest library to engage in the process.

Pointers on Grant Proposal Writing.   Grant proposals may be unsolicited (i.e., you identify a donor and make contact with the individual or agency) or solicited via a request for application (RFA), Request for Statement of Capability (RSC), or a Request for Proposal (RFP). In any case, the basic funding proposal should include eight major elements: cover sheet or title page, abstract or summary of proposal, statement of problem or need, specific aims or objectives of project, methodology, facilities and personnel, budget, and supporting documentation. Permission has been granted by Patricia L. Thibodeau, Duke University Medical Center Library to include the following grant-writing tips:

Title page. The title page should include the project title, name and title of principal investigator, name and address of your institution, the type of grant, name and/or number of the specific funds being sought, and the date.

Abstract. The abstract is usually one paragraph, less than half a page long. The summary should state the purpose of the project, why it is needed, what benefits will be gained, the objectives of the project, and how they will be accomplished (methodology). The abstract provides reviewers with a quick overview of the project and sells your idea, so make sure it is concise, clear, and readable.

Statement of the problem. In the statement of the problem, explain why the project is needed and whom it will benefit. You may want to discuss the history of the situation, note statistical and factual data, review the literature, and quote other appropriate sources. Remember, this is your chance to tell them why the project is so important and must be funded. Additional information that may help the reviewer could include: description of the institutions involved, their mission and prior successes, unique features of the geographic region, population or socioeconomic factors, and state, regional, or local initiatives that this proposal supports or supplements.

Aims or objectives. When detailing aims and objectives of the project, state exactly what you plan to accomplish. Be very specific and make sure the objectives can be measured. For example: Teach 10 regional classes; increase attendance by 10 percent; reduce incidence of x by 5 percent. Make your goals realistic and achievable.

Methodology. The section on methodology should describe in a realistic manner how you will achieve each of your aims and objectives. Be sure to include a time line that lists the major steps in achieving your objectives. The time line can be stated in months or quarters, and can be done in the form of a narrative or a chart. Make sure to address data collection: the tools for collecting the data, how often the data will be collected, and how it will be analyzed. Discuss who will be responsible for accomplishing these tasks: the principal investigator, a new staff person, expert in the field, consultant, and/or other.

Facilities and personnel. When addressing facilities and personnel, discuss the resources—personnel, equipment, space, and so on—needed to accomplish the project. Justify why existing staff and the principal investigator are qualified to manage and implement this project. A brief biographical sketch highlighting pertinent skills and expertise of all key personnel should be included. Explain why additional staff is needed, their responsibilities and required qualifications. Equipment can range from a desk to a car to a high-powered computer system, so it is necessary to explain why it is needed in terms of the objectives and purposes of the project. Do not overlook space considerations: where the staff and project will be housed, what additional space or renovations to space will be needed, and where the facility is located.

Budget presentation. Line-item is the preferred style of budget presentation. Key staff and new positions should be listed individually. Otherwise, the traditional categories of Personnel, Equipment, Supplies, Travel, and Other Expenses can be used. Each of these can be broken down into more detailed categories if it is felt to be necessary. The larger the request, the more detail you should provide. One tip is to provide a summary budget sheet using only the broad line-item categories, and then place the more detailed budget information following it. Very detailed information such as the specifications and costs of each component of a major computer system could be placed in the appendices. If you are not requesting funds for staff, space, equipment, and so on, you can show this as "in-kind" support in the budget or narrative.

Supporting documents and detailed information. This information should be placed in the appendices. This makes the proposal easy to read while ensuring that the more specific information is available to the reviewers. Letters of support from collaborating agencies, statewide agencies, constituents who will benefit from the project, and other key people and institutions help strengthen your proposal and show community support. Maps quickly summarize the area and impact of the project. Diagrams, charts, and illustrations should be used if they are clear and effective and support key points in the document. Curriculum vitae for key personnel should be included. Annual reports are required in some cases. Also, bids from suppliers for various planned purchases can be included.

Proposed elements. Make sure the elements of the proposal all tie together. If you put a computer in your budget, make sure you include it in your methodology and in your description of facilities. Do not ask for personnel and never explain what they will be doing. Tie together your objectives, methodology, resources, and budget.

Reporting requirements. Once you are funded, make sure that you know what the reporting requirements are, the frequency of written reports, and the type of budget and reimbursement forms to be used. There may also be other requirements and restrictions that you need to make it your business to be aware of, including official signatures and final forms.

Sources of Information on Grants

For the most comprehensive collection of grants resources, visit the Foundation Center Web site at http://fdncenter.org. Additional sources are included in the Suggested Readings for this chapter.

PERSONNEL MANAGEMENT

Nothing is more important to a library than the quality of the staff. Good staff can often compensate for limited funds by making exceptional use of the available resources; but extensive (or expensive) collections will not compensate for untrained or disinterested staff. "A good organization trains its employees to do their jobs well, gives them the knowledge to function successfully, and instills in them a commitment to their work" (Blocklyn, 1988, p. 35).

Types of Library Staff and Functions

The basic characteristics most important in selecting nursing library personnel are: commitment to service, flexibility in the face of rapid change, and a curiosity that results in the pursuit of new knowledge and skills. Staff size and duties are governed by the size of the library and service level desired. Academic libraries have larger staffs, with specialized roles, such as cataloging, reference services, or collection management. Hospital libraries or information centers are frequently staffed by only one or two individuals, usually a professional librarian and a technical assistant, but sometimes by only a nondegreed library manager. In these smaller libraries or centers, all operations must be handled by the limited staff or contracted out.

Typical Library Activities and Job Roles. Basic tasks, or job roles, in a library can include:

- *Administration.* The development and evaluation of policies, goals, and services, including quality assurance; strategic planning; the development and management of budgets; the supervision, education and training, staffing, and scheduling of personnel; the oversight of the library's physical plant; oversight of safety and security measures; reporting on the library's activities and communicating with all levels of the library's service population, from the senior management of the parent organization to the everyday library user or student library aide. Administrative duties may also include the development of funding sources or grant proposals.

- *Reference service.* Compilation of bibliographies on specific subjects as requested or for the location of specific answers to inquiries from users, often involving the use of multiple types of sources such as books, online databases, or the Internet; the proactive development of specific tools, files, indexes, or other resources specific to the needs of the institution's users.

- *Collection development and acquisitions.* The selection and purchasing of materials or services for the library. This can include audiovisual materials, CD-ROM databases, journals, or specific online services. In some organizations, the selection and purchasing of services, especially online systems or database materials, is the purview of reference staff. In larger libraries, different staff may be experts in specific subject areas, and thus responsible for the selection of materials in those subjects. In large academic libraries, collection development is often coordinated by one individual who also serves as part of the reference staff, in order to keep in touch with user needs. Collection development duties also include the "weeding," or disposal, of outdated materials in the library's collection and the acknowledgment and handling of gift materials. Good collection development requires familiarity with the programs and health services the library supports, supplemented by up-to-date knowledge and evaluation of the library collection's strengths and weaknesses in relation to changing user needs and requests.

- *Serials management.* The ordering, checking in, claiming, and binding of journals. Even in smaller libraries, journals are usually purchased through an agent, or jobber, who assists in the process of claiming issues that have not been received. Binding is almost always contracted out. Serials may include the handling of periodic publications, such as annual reviews or directories.

- *Document delivery/interlibrary loans.* The provision of requested photocopies of items in the collection, or the loan of materials to outside organizations or individuals (document delivery); the obtaining of materials not available in the collection for users (interlibrary loan). This is a rapidly changing area of library service, and requires knowledge of resource-sharing protocols and networks, of copyright restrictions and regulations, and of new electronic location and delivery methods.

- *Cataloging.* Producing records of items in the library's collection, usually in an online system, using standard classification and subject heading authorities. The result is the ongoing development of a database of the library's holdings. Call number labeling and other such types of end processing may be done by cataloging staff.

- *Circulation/public services.* Checking materials in and out of the library, following up overdue items, maintaining records of the library's eligible borrowers, answering basic directional or informational questions, making change for copy machines, and so on. In larger libraries, this might also include the placement of items on reserve for special classes or programs.

- *Instruction/orientation.* Teaching clientele how to use online databases, the Internet, or reference materials; or, in larger libraries, providing formal or even for-credit instruction on information organization, access, and use, including routine tours and orientations and the development of brochures or educational materials related to the library. Large libraries may staff an educational activities position, but in many libraries, educational duties are performed by reference and public services staff.

- *Collection management.* Shelving, repair of damaged items, and evaluating and addressing space needs for materials. Sometimes, bindery preparation is handled by this position instead of by serials staff.

- *Media/audiovisual services.* This can include the processing and loan of models, computer software, films, videotapes, and so on. In some organizations, this also includes the setup and running of specialized audiovisual equipment, such as videotaping or slide production.

- *Outreach services.* In larger libraries, often an individual is charged with the responsibility of designing and promoting services to user groups identified by the organization as desirable clients. An example would be large academic libraries that include service to rural practitioners as part of their organizational mission.

- *Systems.* The oversight of computer systems, hardware, and software used to support the library's services. In smaller libraries, this support may come from other departments in the parent institution or be contracted out.

Dawn Bick & Deborah Graham

Qualifications. In large libraries, primarily academic institutions, administrative and reference services are performed by librarians with a master's degree in library or information science, obtained from an institution accredited by the American Library Association. Usually, these positions also require several years of experience in a health sciences library. The Medical Library Association can provide suggested job descriptions for many library positions. One can also use the professional library listservs to access position descriptions from other organizations. A significant development in health sciences librarian job descriptions was the requirement of the Joint Commission on Accreditation of Healthcare Organizations (JCAHO) that job descriptions be criteria-based (Koch, 1989). Criteria-based job descriptions contain specific, quantifiable performance measures that can be used to objectively evaluate performance. In larger libraries, senior positions may require or prefer a second advanced degree (such as a master's in nursing) for librarians specializing in particular subject areas or those specializing in service to specific groups, such as distance-education students or rural health care practitioners. It has become increasingly important that health sciences librarians at all levels be well versed in the use of electronic information systems and services.

Expectations, Training, and Evaluation. Few librarians receive substantial supervisory or management training as part of their professional degree, thus the parent institution should ensure that librarians in supervisory positions receive at least a basic course of instruction in fundamentals of personnel management, if for no other reason than the legal protection of the organization. If such support is not available, the librarian should take the initiative to seek out either a mentor or formal instruction. The primary steps of supervision and effective employee development include:

1. *Clear definition of the goals and mission of the library/organization.* If an organization has not defined what it does and why, it is nearly impossible for an employee to develop a sense of commitment and investment in the enterprise. If employees know the

mission of the organization and what their job requires, they can make good decisions on day-to-day matters with less supervision and a greater sense of accomplishment. Communicating mission requires continuous role-modeling and constant vigilance. Organizational or administrative decisions must be consistently in harmony with the mission if employees are to value it. Developing a staff to the level of true participative management requires that all individuals have the information, the organizational philosophical background, and the interpersonal skills to make good group decisions. It is a long and continuous process that begins with engaging an individual's commitment to and enthusiasm about the organization's mission.

2. *Clear definition of individual job roles and on-the-job expectations.* Many personnel problems arise because a supervisor assumes employees know what is expected of them and how to do it. An employee's understanding must be checked and verified. Asking for help either in defining a task or developing new skills to complete it must be encouraged. Basic practices (attendance, sick leave, etc.) must be consistently and uniformly defined within the organization. Employees need solid definition of basic policies and procedures and assurance that good job performance and competence are part of the organizational culture. Performance is highest in organizations where all employees can rely on the competence and commitment of coworkers. Many employers make the erroneous assumption that poor on-the-job attitudes cannot be changed. It is acceptable to make contributions to the cooperative and effective operation of a unit through good interpersonal skills a part of a job description, thereby making it a performance expectation that can and should be appraised and evaluated.

3. *Clear understanding of supervision.* Employees need to know that their supervisor's job, and goal, is to help

them succeed, not to find fault. Supervisors need to realize that, usually, an employee's failure is also their failure. Often, poor performance is the result of unclear direction, insufficient training, or of hiring an individual unskilled for the job—all of which are primarily supervisory errors. On the other hand, there are few rewards as great as seeing an employee develop skills and professional expertise under one's direction and encouragement, and achieve successes they had never dreamed of. Employees cannot work effectively in the absence of honest, frequent feedback. Supervisors can be particularly negligent in "catching people doing something right." An important part of the supervisor's job is acknowledging when employees perform well and rewarding them with recognition that is genuinely deserved.

Staff Development

Identifying useful continuing educational opportunities is not difficult. Several major library associations provide continuing education for librarians: the Medical Library Association, the Special Libraries Association, the American Library Association and its subgroups and sections, the American Medical Informatics Association, and the American Society of Information Scientists. Many of these organizations maintain home pages on the World Wide Web, and most include a calendar of educational events. Many local chapters of these organizations are also on the Web, and the activities of the National Network of Libraries of Medicine (NN/LM), sponsored by the National Library of Medicine are distributed in the central and regional Web home pages. Library personnel should be encouraged to take advantage of courses offered by these associations or by their local chapters. In addition, library personnel should be encouraged to attend job-related conferences as well as programs and exhibits at the annual conventions of regional and national library and information science organizations, to keep abreast of trends and new developments relating to information services, products, and equipment.

The information sciences field is changing rapidly, at an unimagined rate, and constant upgrading of skills is an integral part of the library profession. Libraries should budget at least 10 percent of an employee's time for the continual updating of skills and knowledge and on-the-job exploration of new systems and information tools. Unfortunately, some organizations that do not flinch at paying large maintenance fees for a computer system often fail to provide for the "maintenance" of the most important asset of the library—the staff. Staff development funding is central to a library's ability to function, and should be budgeted accordingly.

In addition to providing for formal educational opportunities and on-the-job practice time, staff development involves keeping staff informed about issues relevant to the parent organization and about changes occurring in the health care professions and delivery systems. In-service education should be scheduled regularly, and be given equal or greater priority as other demands on employee time. Activities that are inexpensive and relatively simple, such as the initiation of journal clubs or the routing of key articles and organizational reports, can communicate the importance of continuous learning and active involvement to staff. Senior library managers must serve as role models and mentors that promote continual intellectual growth, and staff must be encouraged and rewarded for participation in professional associations and educational activities.

Volunteers

Whether a library uses volunteer staff may depend on the parent organization's regulations. There are specific legal issues or liabilities that may make the use of volunteers counterproductive. Hospital libraries traditionally have had access to an official volunteer office and coordinator through their parent organizations, which usually screen applicants for those skills that the librarian has identified as useful. Volunteers should be given the same clear direction as to their job role and duties that is provided to paid staff. If they are not well oriented and trained, it can be excessively time-consuming to find activities for them to do, and they can cause more work for the staff than is justified by the help they give. Volunteers who clearly understand a task, and particularly those who are given a routine project that is theirs alone to handle, can be valuable long-term members of the library team, and should be recognized and treated as such.

Contracting for Services

Contracting out for services, or "outsourcing," has become a trend in smaller libraries attempting to cope with staff reductions, and has long been standard practice for some services, such as binding. The types of service that can be handled by an outside contractor vary with the type and size of the library. Single-person operations may have to contract out even online literature searching in order to provide the level of services desired. Larger libraries may find that new needs resulting from technological changes require skills not available among present staff, but those needs may not be of sufficient volume to justify the addition of actual staff positions. Examples of services that can effectively be contracted out are online literature searching and document delivery/interlibrary loans, cataloging, and binding.

Online Literature Searching. This can be an effective tactic for the manager of a small hospital library, particularly if the library manager has limited experience with multiple databases and additional job duties beyond the care of the library. A larger health sciences library may be able to provide rapid (fax) delivery of literature searches of higher quality, and in cases where online charges accumulate by the minute, less expense, as the experienced searcher can get in and out of a system more efficiently. Some larger health sciences libraries even have searchers who specialize in specific subject areas, providing a level of expertise that simply could not be achieved by a single library manager who has neither the time nor the volume of requests in a specific subject area to become proficient in that field. One commercial database vendor, DIALOG, offers a service that includes the running of subject searches, not just the provision of access to its database systems, as a substitute for vacationing library staff.

Document Delivery/Interlibrary Loans. There are efficient networks designed to facilitate ordering and delivery of copies of articles or the loan of books that a library does not have in its own collection. The existence of online catalogs, and giant fee-for-service article databases (such as CARL/UnCover, which provides access to article citations for over 20,000 journal titles) provide users even in geographically remote communities with access to needed professional literature. In recent months, increasing numbers of professional health sciences journals have appeared on the World Wide Web. Many provide the full text of at least some of the articles in an issue at no charge. As additional organizations publish their materials online, professional literature should become both more accessible and less costly.

Libraries are examining the cost of maintaining on-site personnel to provide document delivery services versus the prices charged by document delivery vendors and the options available through new technologies. Vendors are designing ever-more sophisticated services, such as UnCover's REVEAL service, which automatically routes tables of contents to users via e-mail when the citations of a new journal issue are added to the database (albeit for a price).

Given the breadth and sophistication of some of these emerging services, they may well be superior alternatives to in-house systems, especially for smaller libraries with few staff. FirstSearch's FASTDOC provides instant full-text access to some titles on the FirstSearch system, a real boon to distance-education students. Such systems can match or reduce the cost of staff-mediated document delivery while improving user satisfaction by providing almost, or actual, immediate access to articles.

Cataloging. National services or larger health sciences libraries in the immediate geographic area can be sources of catalog records. Pitfalls in contracting for this service include the loss of "local" value-adding enhancements to records and the difficulty of dealing with system compatibilities. Catalogs and catalog services on the national level use the MARC (Machine-Readable Cataloging records) format. While this is an industry standard that is widely accepted and honored, some very small libraries may find the cost of obtaining MARC records and of maintaining systems capable of using them to be greater than the benefit received. In larger libraries, almost all cataloging is done through the Online Computer Library Center, Inc. (OCLC) system, the major contractor for cataloging records. OCLC also serves as a locating service for interlibrary loans and provides a searchable article database system, FirstSearch. FirstSearch subscribers who also use OCLC for cataloging can have citations of locally owned journal titles identified for end users, a considerable time-saver.

Binding. This service is almost always contracted out, as the specialized equipment required would not make in-house binding of journals cost-effective. Very small libraries that choose to keep five years or less of a journal title may decide not to bind materials.

In selecting contractors, it is critical to have information about them from other libraries. Listservs are particularly good for inquiring about possible vendors of a specific service, and for checking on their reputation and performance record within the professional library community.

Advertisements in professional journals are another source for identifying potential service providers, and most now have home pages on the World Wide Web. Major services, such as online article database systems or major online catalog companies will have been written about in articles in professional information sciences journals, either specifically or as part of more global reviews that provide comparative evaluations of vendors for specific types of services. One final word of caution: Never do business with an agent or company that you do not feel good about. Instinct is often as valuable as information, and a good working relationship is critical to effective vendor-client results, particularly when crises arise. If you do not feel confident and comfortable with a vendor, investigate another option.

Consultants

Every library at one time or another requires the assistance of a specialist in an area of expertise that is not available from the library's staff or the parent institution, in which case consultants can be particularly useful in helping libraries attempting major changes in service directions or organizational structure. Individuals outside an organization can often spot barriers to service (quite literally, as in assessing traffic patterns in a service desk area) that staff are no longer able to see because of habit or the pressures of day-to-day operations. Sometimes, the installation of new hardware and software systems requires training that can best be provided by outside experts. The initiation of major new services or design of a new building will almost certainly involve the use of field-specific experts. Professional journals often list consultants in a variety of fields. Another method of identifying consultants is to search the World Wide Web or broadcast an inquiry to professional listservs. Consultants are available for every conceivable library activity. As with contractors, it is essential to check references and investigate the track record of a consultant before committing to a contract for services. Some organizations require specific procedures (such as a bidding process) for the use of either contractors or consultants, and the library must adhere to these requirements. Joseph Matthews has written a comprehensive review on use of consultants in libraries, which includes samples of library-consultant agreements. Any library considering the use of a consultant will find a review of his article useful (Matthews, 1994).

Consultants usually charge by the hour or day. Do not waste their time or the library's money. Spell out the desired goal of a consultation clearly so they can request any documents needed for review or schedule appointments with key staff members in advance. Specify exactly what you expect them to furnish as a result of the consultation, such as written reports or presentations. For example, smaller libraries may want a consultation on the adequacy or design of their services, particularly as a prelude to accreditation site visits. If library staff members have a good working relationship with professionals in larger libraries in the area, they might do well simply to ask for assistance from colleagues known to them. Regional and resource libraries of the National Network of Libraries of Medicine, discussed in Chapter 10, have as part of their mission the commitment to assist smaller libraries, and may themselves provide consultant services or sound advice about a wide range of library issues. Contact one of these resources before deciding whether bringing in a consultant is necessary and worth the price.

PUBLIC RELATIONS

Marketing the Library and Its Services

Marketing strategies and activities for library and information services are specific to the user group, or "market," one is trying to reach. Good marketing consists of: the identification, or creation, of user (customer) needs; and the ongoing design or development of services or products that meet those needs.

Marketing of the library and its services should not be done to promote what users *should* want. Neither should marketing be done to sell services or products for their own sake or to generate revenue. Good marketing is always client-centered; that is, the user/customer must experience genuine "value received" from every transaction; it must be sufficiently useful or desirable to justify the cost to them either in dollars, or, if no fees are involved, in time. Ideally, services and products should exceed user/customer expectations, and those responsible for products and services should continually monitor client satisfaction levels. Marketing then becomes a process of continuous self-evaluation and strategic service development that will ensure the recognition of the library's value to its clients. In an era of cost-cutting and containment, skilled marketing is essential to a library's survival.

The first step in developing a marketing strategy is to take the time to analyze the audiences or markets, or client base, one is trying to reach. There may be primary and secondary client groups or markets; for example, an academic nursing library has as its primary clientele the faculty and students of the school, but it may also actively serve professional nurses in the community, a secondary market. Once markets are identified and prioritized, specific services or "products" can be identified that are of particular importance to the markets. Sometimes it is possible to develop actual "product lines," such as a variety of online bibliographic search services or specific document delivery services that will fit the needs of several groups, while meeting the needs specific to each one.

All services have an existing market—the individuals who use the service. By examining how current users perceive the service, one can better determine improvements to implement in existing services or more effectively identify new services that fulfill unmet needs. Examination of how existing clients are actually using services, and what unmet needs they have, is referred to as a "marketing audit" (Bunyan & Lutz, 1991). Such audits can include the collection of data from routine contacts, statistics on daily activities, and surveys or questionnaires. The object is to identify user needs, barriers to meeting those needs, and strategies for successfully fulfilling unmet needs within personnel and budget limitations. A marketing orientation implies a commitment to continually evaluate costs of activities and the benefits, or degree of user satisfaction, resulting from those activities. This shift in perception can result in innovative new services, refinement, or discontinuation of established services. User satisfaction, ideally "delight," with services received becomes the primary focus around which the library's activities are designed and evaluated.

An example of the marketing process follows. The librarian feels that a service to alert nursing supervisors to new books or journal articles of high relevance to them would be worthwhile. The first step in the process would be to verify that this is indeed a service the nurses would use. (Ask: Is there really a need?) Sometimes a market can be "created" at this step in the process; by bringing the idea of a service to the attention of potential users, it generates a perceived need where none had existed. Once the need for the service is validated (using marketing audit techniques) the next step is to design the service so it is as easy to use as possible. In this case, the librarian may have identified a process of posting announcements on the library's electronic bulletin board or World Wide Web home page as a rapid and cost-effective approach. But if the nurses do not have convenient access to computers capable of accessing the library's bulletin board or home page, the service will be useless. If the targeted audience can access the announcements, can they also get away from the patient care areas to check out or use the materials?

Too often, libraries have stopped at the point of informing users about resources or services, and considered their marketing or promotional duties done. Any promotion or marketing of services must have as its goal the successful use of information resources. Product design must therefore include solutions to any problems or barriers that might prevent effective use of a service. As health care professionals, nurses have significant barriers to using library or information services (Royle, Blythe, Potvin, Oolup, & Chan, 1995), including increased productivity goals in health care facilities, longer shifts, and personal time demands that make access during library hours difficult. Other barriers include lack of equipment for electronic access to databases or Internet resources or fees for interlibrary loan requests. The librarian must investigate exactly how a service will function as part of the design process. The solution may require posting announcements in multiple places (e.g., the nursing staff newsletter, on the unit bulletin boards, or in electronic formats) and even instituting a delivery service to make actual use of materials possible.

Consider carefully before initiating any new service. Be sure that personnel and financial resources are available, or that pricing is accurate and viable. It is essential to avoid raising expectations that cannot be met, a situation referred to as "overpromising and underdelivering."

Promoting the Library and Its Services

A library should be dynamic, constantly improving the quality and usefulness of its services. But even service excellence cannot guarantee that a library will receive the institutional or user recognition essential to its survival. In order to promote library services, the librarian must be aware of key goals and programs of the parent organization, and design marketing activities that proactively support those programs and goals. Activities that can enhance the perception of the library's value to the organization include:

- *Anticipatory literature searches or materials awareness services.* Produce and publicize the availability of bibliographies on subjects of current importance to the parent organization. These can be published in the library's newsletter, made the focus of a special display, or customized for key individuals. Know the interests of important figures in the organization, and alert them to articles of special interest, or provide routine monthly alert services. Conduct ongoing, proactive evaluation of materials in the collection, and proactive purchasing of materials in support of new programs or subject areas. This requires an awareness of organizational and health industry changes and activities beyond the library's walls.

- *Visibility.* The librarian, or different members of the library staff should participate in committees or events that cross organizational/departmental lines. This can be as simple as offering to help with a United Way campaign or as complex as actively participating on a practice guidelines or curriculum committee. Advantage should be taken of any open invitations to participate in organizational information fairs or other events that promote specific departments or services.

- *Advertising.* Use traditional advertising approaches, such as "table tents," posters, brochures, and bookmarks. The American Library Association has a catalog of promotional materials, and other library groups such as the Medical Library Association or Special Libraries Association also produce promotional materials.

- *Informational materials and newsletters.* The library should have some mechanism of announcing new materials and services; and a library newsletter, even if only quarterly, is achievable by most libraries. If possible, have regular columns in other department newsletters (nursing, pharmacy, etc.). Printed materials or electronic resource pages sponsored by the library should be reviewed periodically for clarity, absence of professional jargon, and for visual appeal. In the case of World Wide Web home pages, links to other resources must be checked at least monthly, so users are not consistently led to expired sources. In an age when many users "come to" the library electronically, it is important to have well-prepared user instruction and help sheets available electronically, as Web pages. This is one way to maintain the availability of the librarian's assistance in cyberspace.

- *Consistent attention to user-friendly service.* This may seem to be a given, but often overlooked are such administrative activities as routine updating of library signage and examination of the physical plant. Maintaining basic personnel principles is critical, including periodically reviewing staffing schedules (ensuring that professional librarians are available when needed) and adjusting hours of service if needed. Procedures and policies should be clear, consistently followed, and reasonable. Staff should be well trained and familiar with the organization's goals, philosophy, and overall operations so they can respond to user needs or inquiries without routinely having to refer users to other staff, or so they can refer accurately and gracefully when necessary. If the library provides orientations or classes, these should be periodically reviewed, evaluated, and revised to reflect changing needs and services. Staff members who provide classes or orientations should be well trained, and have access to educational resources so their presentation skills are up to date. If at all possible, phone inquiries should be answered by a person, not a machine. Voice mail and automated phone systems have been widely employed in many service organizations, but they are far from user-friendly. In an era when increasingly large amounts of data and information can be accessed directly by individuals, without the assistance of the library, the survival of libraries may well depend upon how well users feel they are being served. A reputation for exceptional service—positive word of mouth among a library's users—is the single most powerful promotional tool available.

Developing Support Groups

Libraries need advocates. These can be repeat, satisfied users who are willing to speak up for funding when needed, or they can be members of advisory committees who help plan new services and evaluate ongoing activities. Many libraries have a "friends" group, which individuals or corporations can join for a specific contribution. Friends of the Library groups may hold fund-raising activities, special events such as book sales or signing parties, and can be called upon to add their voices and influence in support of funding and their time as volunteers for special on-site events. Fortunately for libraries, many individuals have strong, positive feelings for libraries in general, and often for a particular library that was important to them during their education or career. With financial resources growing ever tighter, libraries will need to engage in fund-raising development activities. A friends group can be a good start. The librarian will need to check with the development office of the parent organization before initiating such activities, in order to set up specific accounts for donations, which are often tax-deductible, and to avoid conflicting with the parent organization's overall development plans. Professional development officers can also advise the librarian about ways to recognize supporters and acknowledge their contributions.

Public Relations: The Bottom Line

Every encounter between users and a library is a public relations encounter. There is the potential for positive enhancement of the

95

library's image and usefulness and conversely, for permanent user disillusionment and resentment. An encounter need not be an interaction between library staff and a user; it may be the interaction with an online catalog or bibliographic search system, or that a user cannot determine where things are in the building without asking for help, or that books are not reshelved accurately and are consistently hard to find. Public relations begins and ends with a genuine commitment to user service as the driving force of the library, and to routine, accurate, and quality performance by all staff. All staff, all systems, all activities must be weighed and evaluated as successful or not in view of that commitment. Promotional materials, publicity, and special events will not compensate for failed public relations in day-to-day operations. Innovative services that promise much but deliver little may look impressive in an organizational publications list but will not deceive those who really use the library. Every staff member of a library has the power to create a positive or negative interaction, either through direct interaction, such as a service desk inquiry, or through the quality of their work, such as a photocopy that is stapled with several pages upside down, or an online system that frequently goes down without warning. It is the head librarian's job to impress upon all staff the importance of their individual efforts, that their individual work or interactions represent the entire library to users. Good public relations begin with good staff training and constant attention to daily operational details, with staff who take pride in and care about their work.

CONCLUSION

This chapter discussed library finance in terms of budget preparation and extensions to the budget in the form of fund-raising and grants. Libraries of all sizes can manage their finances utilizing the basic principles presented. The resourceful library manager can be successful in developing a sound financial base that will enable unique and specialized services to meet the needs of the library's clientele.

The personnel management section detailed the roles, qualifications, and ongoing training of library staff. Finally, the public relations section underlined the importance of delivering high-quality services to users in a consistently positive manner.

REFERENCES

Black, W. K. (1993). The budget as a planning tool. *Journal of Library Administration, 18,* 171–188.

Blocklyn, P. L. (1988). Making magic: The Disney approach to people management. *Personnel, 65,* 28–35.

Bunyan, L. E., & Lutz, E. M. (1991). Marketing the hospital library to nurses. *Bulletin of the Medical Library Association, 79,* 223–225.

Burlingame, D. F. (1994). Fund-raising as a key to the library's future. *Library Trends, 42,* 467–477.

Koch, H. F. (1989). Criteria-based performance evaluations for hospital library managers. *Special Libraries, 80,* 269–274.

Lapsley, A. (1995). The business of corporate giving. *The Bottom Line, 8*(2), 41–44.

Matthews, J. (1994). The effective use of consultants in libraries. *Library Technology Reports, 30,* 745–814.

Nielsen, S. (1992–1993). Ten "quick and dirty" cost-cutting strategies for your library. *The Bottom Line, 6*(2), 40–42.

Robinson, D. M., & Robinson, S. (1994). Strategic planning and program budgeting for libraries. *Library Trends, 42,* 420–447.

Royle, J. A., Blythe, J., Potvin, C., Oolup, P., & Chan, I. M. (1995). Literature search and retrieval in the workplace. *Computers in Nursing, 13,* 25–31.

Sirota, M. (1992). Time is money. *The Bottom Line, 6*(1), 15–18.

Stanley, N. M. (1993). Accrual accounting and library materials acquisitions. *The Bottom Line, 7,* 15–17.

Stoffle, C. J. (1992). The politics of budgeting. *The Bottom Line, 6*(2), 9–16.

Thibodeau, P. L. (1993). *Hints for writing a successful grant proposal.* Unpublished paper.

Tucker, D. C. (1992). Donor research can improve your library's fund-raising efforts. *The Bottom Line, 6*(2), 17–22.

White, H. S. (1992). Seeking outside funding: The right and wrong reasons. *Library Journal, 117,* 48–49.

Dawn Bick & Deborah Graham

RESOURCE REFERENCES

Dolnick, S. (1990). *Friends of the libraries sourcebook*. Chicago: American Library Association.

Lipow, A. G., & Carver, D. A. (Eds.). (1992). *Staff development: A practical guide*. Chicago: American Library Association.

Martin, M. S. (1995). *Collection development and finance: A guide to strategic library-materials budgeting*. Chicago: American Library Association.

McNeil, B., & Johnson, D. J. (1996). *Patron behavior in libraries: A handbook of positive approaches to negative situations*. Chicago: American Library Association.

Prentice, A. E. (1996). *Financial planning for libraries*. Lanham, MD: Scarecrow Press.

Rounds, R. S. (1994). *Basic budgeting practices for librarians*. Chicago: American Library Association.

Rubin, R. (1991). *Human resources management in libraries: Theory and practice*. New York: Neal-Schuman.

Sager, D. J. (1992). *Small libraries: Organization and operation*. Fort Atkinson, WI: Highsmith Press.

Smith, G. S. (1991). *Managerial accounting for libraries and other not-for-profit organizations*. Chicago: American Library Association.

Stueart, R. D. (1991). *Performance analysis and appraisal: A how-to-do-it manual for librarians*. New York: Neal-Schuman.

Turock, B. J., & Pedolsky, A. (1992). *Creating a financial plan: A how-to-do-it manual for librarians*. New York: Neal-Schuman.

Walters, S. (1992). *Marketing: A how-to-do-it manual for librarians*. New York: Neal-Schuman.

SUGGESTED READINGS

Birdsall, D. G. (1995). The micropolitics of budgeting in universities: Lessons for library administrators. *Journal of Academic Librarianship, 21,* 427–437.

Campbell, J. D. (1994). Getting comfortable with change: A new budget model for libraries in transition. *Library Trends, 42,* 448–459.

Christianson, E. (1993). When your parent dictates your accounting life. *The Bottom Line, 7*(2), 17–21.

Christianson, E. B., King, D. E., & Ahrensfeld, J. L. (1991). *Special libraries: A guide for management*. Chicago: Special Libraries Association.

Cram, L. (1995). The marketing audit: Baseline for action. *Library Trends, 43,* 326–348.

Dunn, J. A., Jr., & Martin, M. S. (1994). The whole cost of libraries. *Library Trends, 42,* 564–578.

Gordon, M. (1994). Accommodating institutional audit requirements within a liberal arts college integrated library system. *Library Acquisitions: Practice & Theory, 18,* 341–350.

Hayes, S., & Brown, D. (1994). The library as a business: Mapping the pervasiveness of financial relationships in today's library. *Library Trends, 42,* 404–419.

Interagency Council on Information Resources for Nursing. (1996). Essential nursing references. *N&HC: Perspectives on Community, 17,* 258.

Kathman, M. D., & Kathman, J. M. (1995). *Managing student library employees: A workshop for supervisors.* Berkeley, CA: Library Solutions Press.

Kratz, C. E., & Platz, V. A. (Eds.). (1993). *The personnel manual: An outline for libraries.* Chicago: American Library Association.

Mackey, T., & Mackey, K. (1992). Think quality! The Deming approach does work in libraries. *Library Journal, 117*(9), 57–61.

Martin, M. S. (1995). Fiscal currents. Gifts, grants and libraries. *The Bottom Line,8*(2), 37–39.

McCarthy, C. A. (1996). Volunteers and technology: The new reality. *American Libraries, 27*(6), 67–73

St. Clair, G., & Williamson, J. (1992). *Managing the new one-person library.* London: Bowker Saur.

Stern, G. J. (1990). *Marketing workbook for nonprofit organizations.* St. Paul, MN: Amherst H. Wilder Foundation.

4

Information and Educational Services

Juliette Ratner, MS
Jacqueline Picciano, MSLS, MBA, FMLA, AHIP
Madeline Turkeltaub, RN, PhD, CRNP

Teaching, research, and practice are generally considered the trifold mission of schools of nursing, although the focus may differ among schools. These three elements are also incorporated into expectations of current nursing practice, which emphasizes the importance of individual nurses in clinical practice, education, and administration having access to and assistance with the ever-increasing body of information resources.

Knowing how to access information and use educational services offered by the library or resource center is a skill as important to nursing today as taking vital signs. The library or resource center is not only considered integral to the nursing school curriculum, but is also regarded as an essential resource for current information applicable to clinical practice. This chapter focuses on nursing information services and their management, whether in a separate nursing library, an integrated library serving nurses, in addition to others.

REFERENCE POLICIES

Reference policies should facilitate the provision of information services tailored to the needs of its primary clientele—be it for faculty and students of the school, an educational program it serves, or staff of a health care center or hospital unit—as determined by the mission of the parent organization and as defined in the overall policy statement of the library. The primary purpose of reference policies is to ensure optimum use of the library's collection and services, therefore each library must determine the policy that keeps it focused on its goals. (General library policies are discussed in Chapter 2.) Reference policies should be in writing, and state what services are available to primary clientele and whether these services will be extended to others, such as alumni, nurses, and other health professionals in the institution, or to patients or the general public. The size of the staff and available resources may determine whether access and information services will be extended to outsiders. Services to outsiders may be limited to use of the existing collection with a minimum of guidance, or broader services may be considered a part of the library's role. If establishing good community relations is a goal, then service to the public may be encouraged, in which case, the library will have to extend the collection and services to include materials and services tailored for their needs.

The librarian who is responsible for reference policies should report to the director of the nursing school, and in many instances, be an active member of a planned program of studies committee, an education committee, or a library committee, which give input to library policy. If the policies are for a school or program of nursing, a student representative should be chosen to represent the student body on the committee. Suggested information to include in a reference policy statement is given in the Appendix at the end of this chapter.

A systematic plan of operation outlines operational techniques and procedures by which to implement the activities of the nursing program in accordance with the philosophy and objectives of the program. As a component of this plan, the library promotes learning and assists in fulfilling the curriculum objectives. Functions to include under reference policies include: reviewing and evaluating library books, periodicals, hardware, software, and other library materials for acquisition and removal by faculty, with the advisement of the librarian and in accordance with the collection and deletion policies; reporting statistics to a planned program of studies committee or library committee enumerating acquisitions, removals, and other library matters; and evaluating library services using a questionnaire (Mountainside Hospital School of Nursing, 1997, p. 15).

PROVIDING REFERENCE AND INFORMATION SERVICES

Reference services may be defined as assistance given by library staff to library clientele seeking information. In most libraries, a reference desk serves as the command post for all users' services. In a one-person library, the librarian's desk will often be an all-purpose workstation and the first point of access for circulation, reference, interlibrary loan, and all other services. In larger libraries, while the reference desk is often separate from the circulation desk, there is a growing trend to have one desk serve as the first contact point. The person at the desk makes the initial contact and refers questions to others when appropriate.

The Reference Interview

The first step in information retrieval is the reference interview, still an important function, even though forms of information retrieval are changing. It consists of a one-on-one communication between the user and the reference librarian, either at the reference desk or over the telephone. If the request reaches the librarian electronically, it will probably be necessary for the librarian to contact the user to clarify it. During the reference interview, the librarian helps the user define his or her question clearly, so that both librarian and user understand exactly what information, why, and how much is needed to meet the request. According to Taylor (1968), there are five filters through which a request passes as the librarian translates it into a searchable question:

103

1. Determination of the subject.
2. Objective and motivation—why information is needed.
3. Personal characteristics of the inquirer.
4. Relationship of the inquiry to resources at hand.
5. Anticipated or acceptable answers.

Library Orientation and Instruction

Orientation. A library orientation program enables the librarian to give an overview of library policies, services, and resources. Library orientations can vary in both quality and level, from merely handing out a general brochure on the library and its services to offering a combination of lectures, brochures on specific services and topics, and a tour. If the library has an online public access catalog (OPAC), a demonstration on usage should be included, along with additional instruction provided on a routine schedule.

Items specifically mentioned during library orientation should include information on:

Eating policy (Allowed, disallowed, tolerated?).

Borrowing privileges (Who are the clientele?).

Reserve section.

Copying policies.

Overdue materials (Where can materials can be returned? Are there fines, penalties?).

Hours (What are the librarian's hours? Is there other coverage? Nights? Weekends?).

Collection (Size? Scope).

Services, for example, interlibrary loan.

Charges and fees, for example, for mediated computer searches.

User guides prepared for orientation should be revised and updated on a regular basis and be distributed during library orientations and to new students and staff, as well as be readily available at all other times in libraries of all sizes. They should provide a brief statement of policies, an explanation of the types and levels of services offered, hours of service, a history of the library, and an overview of the collection. They should also include a list of nursing journals, indexes and abstracts; note special collections; describe equipment available, along with fees, if any; and list staff members with their telephone numbers. Ideally, these guides should promote independent use of the library's resources.

Instruction. Library instruction must be carried out on an ongoing basis and on a variety of levels. It is the key to encouraging independent use of library and information resources, possibly for lifelong learning. Although printed library instructional research guides abound, including one specifically targeting nurses (Strauch, Linton, & Cohen, 1992), and guides to the literature such as that by Schockley (1988), a study revealed that many students and nurses are unaware of the scope of nursing literature and how to access it (Blythe, Royle, Oolup, Potvin, & Smith, 1995). In addition, Spath and Buttlar (1996) found in a survey conducted at Kent State University, Ohio, that only 4 percent of nurses used the library to keep abreast of new developments in the field.

If the curriculum permits, the ideal way to familiarize students with the nursing literature is to offer sessions in the classroom in conjunction with assigning written research projects (Tylor & Switzer, 1991). If this is not possible, the librarian can schedule formal or informal classes. Larger libraries with more reference/instruction librarians may offer a more elaborate range of courses, such as use of the catalog or database searching and advanced practice sessions for specific databases. Certainly, if the library has Internet access, classes on the Internet should be offered, emphasizing biomedical resources on the World Wide Web (the Web).

Further, custom-tailored courses can be developed for specific groups upon request and possibly incorporated into the curriculum. Topics for these courses may include the use of specific software applications, concepts of information management, using the Internet, database searching, updates on new materials in the library, or information access and management. According to Silverstein (1995), students and library clientele expect technology to improve access to information and service, but unless they are taught how to take advantage of these resources, they will become frustrated in their research efforts and/or overburden the library staff with need for guidance.

No wonder the education of end users is now a major component of information services. Teaching can be done on a one-on-one basis or in organized classes, and should include new faculty members (whose instruction should be conducted at a time convenient to their schedules), graduate students, and staff nurses conducting research for undergraduate or graduate courses or to meet certification requirements.

A half-hour in a classroom is often enough to offer a brief overview geared to the computer neophyte, supplemented with individual instruction at the workstation. The format can be adapted to each group's needs. Tyler found that a growth in student competence was observed when they received instruction on basic library skills in a supportive environment, followed by a tour of the library and hands-on experience (Tyler & Switzer, 1991).

Reference Resources

In order to provide information services for nurses, a nursing library will need basic general reference works (dictionaries, a good encyclopedia, and directories of various kinds, including telephone books, zip code directories, and directories of social agencies) as well as specific medical and nursing references. If, however, a nursing school is part of a university, or if students and faculty have access to public or college or university libraries containing these general reference resources, they need not be duplicated in the nursing library. Standard biomedical resources, including MEDLINE and the *Index Medicus* still will be needed unless the nursing library is an integral part of a medical library or the students have access to one.

"Essential Reference Sources" (Interagency Council on Information Resources for Nursing, 1996) is a list of basic reference materials that can be used in setting up a nursing collection. Revised every two years, it includes both the general and biomedical resources necessary for nursing information retrieval and those specifically nursing-oriented. Its range includes teaching, research, administration, histories, indexes and abstracts, legal guides, and writers' manuals, as well as audiovisuals and computerized databases.

The Brandon nursing list is another excellent tool for developing a collection, especially for those librarians not familiar with nursing literature (Brandon & Hill, 1996). But is not intended to cover reference books. In a small nursing library, however, textbooks may become reference books and may be displayed on the reference shelf. Publishers' catalogs also can be useful in identifying reference books to include in a nursing collection. The names and addresses of most of the major publishers of nursing materials are listed in the printed version of the *Cumulative Index to Nursing & Allied Health Literature* (CINAHL). Finally, *Doody's Nursing and Allied Health Review Quarterly*, discussed in Chapter 5, reviews publications suitable for reference services. Additional reference sources are included at the end of this chapter.

Electronic Databases. Even the smallest nursing library will need access to databases, either online or on CD-ROM; and in particular, access to MEDLINE and CINAHL is essential. MEDLINE provides access to citations from about 3,700 biomedical journals including citations to articles in all the nursing journals indexed for the *International Nursing Index*. CINAHL lists citations to information from some 800 journals on nursing, allied health, and various consumer health and library literature.

Other databases to be considered are HealthSTAR, covering health services, administration, technology, administration and research; RNdex, a new index covering the top 100 nursing research journals; PsycINFO, for psychology; ERIC, for education; and Current Contents from the Institute for Scientific Information, which indexes recent tables of contents from journal issues. Consumer-oriented databases should also be evaluated for inclusion.

Because more users today want to do their own database searching, in recent years the nursing library has been challenged to provide end user access to automated search systems. In networked databases, faculty, staff, and students may be able to search them from home or from their office computers. LAN, WAN, and CD-ROM setups in the library, as discussed in Chapter 2, enable convenient access to databases and other online services by multiple end users at a fixed cost, without limiting the number of searches performed on the system at the same time. However, as Cibbarelli, Gertel, and Kratzert (1993) point out, choosing the appropriate format and medium to use to provide access to electronic resources requires careful research and evaluation of the many new products available in the technology, from print, CD-ROM, online, microform, or locally mounted databases. Each format has specific issues associated with costs, time limits on data currency, and information transfer, all of which must be considered by the librarian.

The librarian should also become knowledgeable about services offered by the various vendors for end-user searching in order to make appropriate referrals. In addition to the end-user search services and document delivery offered by the NLM via Grateful Med, discussed in Chapter 10, other such services include:

- CINAHLdirect, provided by Cinahl Information Systems. Document delivery is available. For additional information, call 1-800-959-7167 or go to the Web site at http://www.cinahl.com.
- The FirstSearch® service, provided by OCLC, permits Internet, dial, or OCLC multidrop-line access to almost 50 databases as well as document delivery. For additional information, telephone 1-800-848-5878, ext. 6251, or visit the Web site at http://www.oclc.org.
- Ovid Online provides access to as many as 83 databases, including the Combined Health Information Database (CHID) through several interfaces. For additional information telephone 1-800-950-2035 or visit the Web site at http://www.ovid.com.
- KR ScienceBase, provided by Knight-Ridder Information, Inc., provides access to about 65 databases, many of which focus on chemical, pharmaceutical, and

biotechnology information. For additional information, telephone 1-800-334-2564 or go to the Web site at http://www.krinfo.com.

In the face of all the new technology that encourages individual research capabilities, it is important to remember that not everyone will want to do their own computer searches. The librarian still will be called upon to conduct work-related searches for nurses and other staff members, with or without a fee, depending upon library policies. Thus, as a minimum, the nursing school library or information center should provide mediated searches for CINAHL and the MEDLINE databases, which are available online. CINAHL and some of the NLM databases are also available on CD-ROM. Many other databases of interest to nurses are listed in the Resource References at the end of this chapter.

One final note on this developing area of information retrieval: Because of space and cost limitations, the trend or temptation is to discard print indexes and rely on computerized resources, but print indexes can prove to be valuable backups for online resources. Those in the nursing field include the *Cumulative Index to Nursing and Allied Health Literature*, the *International Nursing Index*, the *Index Medicus*, and the *Hospital and Health Administration Index*.

Government and Association Publications

This publication category includes reports of task forces, vital statistics, health care policy, epidemiology, and legislation. Those of interest to nurses are listed by the issuing agency or organization in the back sections of the print version of the *International Nursing Index*.

Government Publications. Depository libraries, excellent sources of government-issued publications, have been set up in most regions. They receive all government documents without cost, and warehouse and organize them for public use and information. A list of these depositories is available from the Superintendent of

Documents, Government Printing Office (GPO), Washington, DC. The Superintendent of Documents classification scheme (SuDoc) may be used as a system for shelving these publications.

In addition to receiving documents from depository libraries on interlibrary loan, material can be often obtained without cost from the issuing agencies or purchased from the Government Printing Office. And state, county, and local health-related information is available from appropriate government agencies. Consult the government section of the local telephone directory for contact information.

Government information is also readily available on the Web sites of the various federal agencies, or from the GPO *Monthly Catalog,* available both in print and online. Lamont (1996) indicates that government health information available in CD-ROM format is listed in the *CD-ROM Compendium* issued by the SIGCAT (Special Interest Group) Foundation on CD-ROM Applications and Technology. Many of these discs, which are often less expensive than the print version of the publication, are available from the U. S. Government Printing Office and the National Technical Information Service (NTIS).

Government information is also available in:

- Legi-Slate, a database that provides information on Congressional proceedings and publications including information on health issues (Wood, 1995).
- The CD-ROM Directory, produced by TFPL Multimedia, lists commercial CD-ROMs in addition to those from the Government Printing Office.

National Nursing Organizations. Publications of the American Nurses Association (ANA) and the National League for Nursing (NLN) numbered series are indexed in both the *International Nursing Index* and CINAHL. Many of these publications should be included in nursing collections because they include position statements, directories, standards, statistics, and other information of value to nurses, usually filed by publication number.

Any publications focused on standards of practice and guidelines by various specialty organizations, such as those developed

110

by the ANA, should be obtained in a timely manner. New, revised, and updated standards are as essential as the versions they replace. It is important to note on a standard and on the catalog record that it has been updated.

It is recommended that nursing libraries take advantage of the option many organizational publishers offer of placing standing orders for publications. This service assures that no issues of publications are missed, thereby keeping the collection up to date. Information on specialty nursing organizations that produce publications is included in Chapter 5.

Grants. Grants are awarded to individuals or groups by foundations and corporations for research. They can take the form of stipends for training or travel, or provide funds for construction or equipment; and when government agencies are the awarding bodies, they may also be in the form of contracts. One of the largest charitable trusts devoted exclusively to excellence in nursing education is the Helene Fuld Health Trust established in 1935, whose purpose is "the improvement of the health, education, and welfare of student nurses" (McAfooes, 1995, p. 2). It awards grants to schools of nursing conferring a license or degree, and are for specific projects or programs. These awards are not given to individuals.

A comprehensive listing of grant resources in the form of directories, periodicals, handbooks, and online databases can be found in the "Essential Nursing Resources" (Interagency Council on Information Resources for Nursing, 1996, p. 258). Government agencies that offer grants to nurses include: the NIH National Institute of Nursing Research at 301-496-0207 or http://www.nih.gov/ninr/; and the Division of Nursing, Bureau of Health Professions, Health Resources and Services Administration, DHHS at 301-443-6193 or http://www.dhhs.gov. Furthermore, the Computer Retrieval of Information on Scientific Projects (CRISP) database provides information on research projects funded by all U. S. Public Health agencies, including the National Institute of Nursing Research. Access http://www.nih.gov /grants/crisp/html or the NIH gopher. It is also available on CD-ROM and through commercial vendors.

Consumer and Patient Education Materials. Library policy will determine how much service to provide to those patients and outsiders who are considered consumers. The Policy Statement of the Consumer and Patient Health Information Section of the Medical Library Association (Medical Library Association, 1996) recognizes the role of the librarian in this process, and defines the role of collection management to include: identification and selection of available resources; building a collection that best meets the needs of the community, and revising the collection on a systematic basis. When the collection includes consumer information publications—such as that by Rees (1994)—and access to databases—such as the Combined Health Information Database (CHID) (Woods, 1996), Health Periodicals Database, or MDX Health Digest (Wehmeyer, 1995)—the world of consumer health information opens to library clientele. CHID consolidates all health promotion and educational materials produced by various federal agencies. MDX is a database that is updated monthly and includes abstracts written in lay terms.

Consumer and patient education materials may be collected selectively depending upon library policies and the needs of primary clientele. Many of these materials are free. For help in this regard, the National Library of Medicine's Directory of Information Resources Online (DIRLINE) provides information on the publications, holdings, and services offered by over 15,000 government agencies, professional societies, self-help groups, and voluntary health organizations. *Health Hotlines,* a booklet that contains a list of the toll-free numbers of organizations in this database, is available free of cost.

When a library is open to the public, staff should be prepared to answer questions on consumer health. Users may be referred to the nursing library by a local public library, hospital medical library, or school library; or they may walk in or telephone. When a collection of patient education materials is maintained, it is useful to evaluate items for reading level, age groups, and languages.

Because nurses advance consumer education and have proven themselves as consistent patient advocates (Canavan, 1996, pp. 1, 8), the Joint Commission on the Accreditation of Healthcare Organizations (JCAHO) standards has increased the focus on

112

consumer information needs. A brief pamphlet on a disease written for the patient or consumer may also provide the kind of general information a student or even a reference librarian needs for background before beginning a search.

The JCAHO's criteria now include a requirement for a patient education committee that reflects interdisciplinary involvement including nurses and a librarian. No doubt, communication regarding the needs of staff nurses, clinical nurse specialists, nurse educators, and nurse practitioners will be included in the discussion of these committees. Using focus groups on the model conducted by the Midcontinental Region of the National Network of Libraries of Medicine (Mullaly-Quijas, Ward, & Woelfl, 1994), will provide specific information about the types of information needed; the point of access, such as in the library, on the unit, or in the ambulatory care setting; and perceived barriers to using the system, including needs for instruction.

Reserve Collections. Reserve collections as differentiated from the reference collection, are generally maintained for the purpose of increasing accessibility to frequently requested materials which, if left in general circulation, would not be available to the many individuals requesting them. Policies regarding maintenance of reserve collections whether books, periodicals, media, software, or a combination of materials—should be clearly communicated and include: who can request that a publication be placed on or removed from the reserve list; how long it is to be kept on reserve; and when it can be taken off reserve.

Reserve collections consist of texts and other materials that must be used in the library because of heavy current demand, such as the latest nursing care plan books in various subject areas, study guides for nursing board exams, audiovisuals, and style manuals. Journal articles listed in a course syllabus as required reading also fall into the reserve category. At the beginning of each semester, the librarian photocopies these articles and files them alphabetically by title, including the journal name and publication date. This procedure deters queuing at the stacks and prevents the dissatisfaction that results when a journal is missing or misfiled.

Materials in reserve collections need to be periodically reviewed, reevaluated, and weeded. When newer editions of reserve materials arrive, their precursors can be placed on circulating shelves.

Extension of Information Services

In addition to providing information services to individual clientele identified in the library reference policy statement, librarians may become proactive and extend their information services to nursing school or hospital committees (for example, information management, patient/family health education, and curriculum committees) so as to more accurately anticipate future needs for resources. In fact, librarians are frequently noted in the nursing program curriculum as those best prepared to share information management strategies. The image of the librarian, and hence the library, is enhanced when the librarian uses special expertise to improve the overall functioning of the institution.

Distance and Extended Campus Library Services (ECLS)

Nursing students not matriculating in the traditional on-campus academic programs, but who are enrolled in external degree, off-campus, extension, upward mobility, part-time, or similar programs also need access to library and information services. Some of these students may not be able to come to the library during regular library hours, thus the library and information services to off-campus or distance-learning programs must address not only the issue of access versus ownership, but also the issue of resources allocated for the provision of services and support for these programs by the parent organization. This is especially significant because accrediting associations more often consider the quality of library services in off-campus programs in the accreditation process (Kascus & Aguilar, 1988; Simmons, 1991). Guidelines for ECLS have been proposed, and are currently undergoing revision, by the American Colleges and Research Libraries Section of the

American Library Association (American Library Association, ACRL, 1990).

EQUIPMENT, FACILITIES, AND FURNISHINGS

Discussion here regarding basic equipment needed to access the collection and provide information services is focused on:

The card catalog and/or automated systems.

The vertical file.

The fax (telefacsimile) machine.

Photocopiers.

The microfilm/microfiche reader/printer.

Additional information on equipment, facilities, and furnishings is included in Chapters 2 and 8.

The Card Catalog

The card catalog is a commonly used physical format for organizing small nursing collections, serving as a locating tool for materials in the library. Usually, each entry is prepared on a 3- by 5-inch card that is filed in a tray in alphabetical order either by author/title or by subject. An alternative is the dictionary catalog with authors, titles, and subjects interfiled alphabetically. Cross-references facilitate locating currently used subjects and forms of names. Guide cards inserted logically throughout the catalog serve as starting points. Each card should include such additional information as appropriate; for example, whether the book is in a "reserve," "reference," "faculty," or other "special category," which may indicate special shelf placement. For additional visual guidance, audiovisual and computer software catalog cards may be color-coded. For standardization, cards should be filed according to the American Library Association Filing Rules (American Library Association, RSTD Filing Committee, 1980), and any local library filing policies that deviate from this standard should be documented.

When cataloging in publication (CIP) information is not readily available for producing catalog cards, as in the case of software and some print materials, the *National Library of Medicine Classification Scheme for the Shelf Arrangement of Materials in the Medical Field and Its Related Sciences* (National Library of Medicine, 1995) and Cutter-Sanborn (Cutter, 1969) are invaluable tools. Chapter 6 has additional information on cataloging.

In the small nursing library, the librarian may continue to do his or her own cataloging without the use of bibliographic utilities like OCLC. Instead, the librarian can produce catalog cards and labels for spines and book pockets by using a software program that conforms to Anglo-American Cataloging Rules (AACR) standards. Features of this type of software program usually include:

Generating continuation cards automatically.

Producing multiple sets of cards.

Printing cards after preview.

Recalling information from disk storage for modification or printing.

Entering information for printing later in batch processing.

Sorting bibliographic reports by author, title, or call number.

In the small library, journals usually are not cataloged; they are accessed through a separate journal list or file, and are shelved alphabetically by title.

In larger libraries, the cataloging and the catalog itself will be automated. This will be discussed further in the section on circulation.

The Vertical File

The vertical file may contain varying materials of value that are ephemeral in nature, odd in format, or not part of the core

116

collection. Therefore, materials may be filed by subject in folders and discarded when no longer relevant. Although time-consuming to update, guides to these files should be provided to facilitate the location of materials. Typical vertical file materials include: patient education pamphlets, newspaper or magazine articles, pictures, and some government publications. In order to remain useful as a reference resource, the vertical file must be weeded on a regular and frequent basis.

The Fax Machine

Telefacsimile has become an essential and cost-effective communication tool. In seconds, it can distribute information interdepartmentally or internationally. If provided as a free service to faculty and administrative staff, it may be located in a secured room to prevent misuse. The fax machine should also be used for interlibrary loans when speed is a major consideration.

Photocopiers

In most libraries, a minimum of two photocopiers—and more, if the library occupies more than one floor—should be provided to eliminate user lines and, hence, disgruntlement, especially since one will frequently be used exclusively for copying interlibrary loan materials. Chapter 8 provides guidance on selecting a photocopier for use in interlibrary loan.

Students usually pay a minimal fee for photocopies, with other users paying a higher rate. If machines are coin-operated, it is important that users be able to make change. In addition, a bypass key should be made available to the librarian, faculty, and student monitors using the copier for library-related tasks. Keeping accurate records is a must for preventing any problems or questions regarding funds collected. In this regard, there may be a copy-counting charge-back arrangement among departments, or prepaid copy cards to increase efficiency. Finally, a fee-based copying service for those who would rather pay than copy may be offered in a library with sufficient staff.

When determining photocopier costs, supplies to factor in include paper, toner and dry ink, and maintenance. Copiers may be purchased outright, leased, or supplied by another department. Some companies provide the aforementioned supplies and maintenance for the privilege of collecting the money accumulated. Maintenance insurance is provided by most companies for a few years after purchase. At the end of this period, service contracts are available and should be seriously considered, as repairs can be very costly.

It is important to post a notice of copyright restrictions near the photocopying machine. A sample is given in Figure 4.1.

NOTICE

Warning Concerning Copyright Restrictions

The copyright law of the United States (Title 17, United States Code) governs the making of photocopies or other reproductions of copyrighted material, including computer software. The person using this equipment is liable for any infringement.

Under certain conditions specified in the law, libraries and archives are authorized to furnish a photocopy or other reproduction. One of these specified conditions is that the photocopy or reproduction is not to be "used for any purpose other than private study, scholarship, or research." If a user makes a request for purposes in excess of "fair use," that user may be liable for copyright infringement.

It is illegal to make copies of the following documents:

United States Bonds	Treasury Notes
Certificates of Deposit	Paper Money
Postal Money Orders	Passports
Draft Registration Cards	Immigration Papers

Figure 4.1   Copyright Notice

Microfilm/Microfiche Readers and Reader-Printers

Because indexes offer retrospective coverage, older articles are being cited with greater frequency, thus librarians must respond to an increased interest in more dated resources. Rather than store back volumes or issues of journals, they may be microfilmed, eliminating the costs of binding, concerns for missing issues, as well as space requirements. The microfilm/microfiche reader and reader-printer provide access to these storage formats. Coin-operated attachments can be installed for revenue-generating operations, with a bypass key available to faculty and staff for work-related use.

CIRCULATION

Circulation Policy

The library's circulation policy should be posted or available at the reference desk. Hours of operation, too, should be posted in a prominent location, with holidays and changes noted prominently. And if student monitors or volunteers work on a regular schedule, their names and hours should be listed so that users know who is in charge at all times. This increases the comfort level when using the facility.

Most items in a school of nursing collection will circulate to faculty and students; in other settings, for example nursing resource centers, materials will usually circulate to those considered primary clientele. When items are checked out, a transaction record is generated, so that they may be located for recall if necessary. Circulation policies usually include: a limit on the number of items one person may borrow; due dates, which may vary for different types of materials; and overdue fines, which should be predetermined and enforced. In the case of book loss or serious damage, it is recommended that the patron be charged the replacement cost, plus 15 percent to cover processing costs. Circulation policy should also clearly state that students who do not return library materials or pay overdue fines may have their grades, diplomas, or transcripts withheld.

Circulation policy generally lists any restricted items, typically the following:

- *Reference materials.* Books and other frequently used items that are to be kept in the library at all times.

- *Reserve materials.* Materials set aside by course instructors and available only to all members of a class, and to be used only in the library.

- *Unusually expensive materials.* Restricted to premises-only use to prevent loss or damage.

- *New and/or unbound periodical issues.* Not available for circulation; available in the library for reading or photocopying only.

- *Bound or unbound periodicals.* Some libraries restrict circulation of all periodicals, bound or not; some libraries do not bind periodicals.

- *Archival materials.* Items important to the institution's history, often irreplaceable.

- *Old or damaged materials.* Used on premises only to prevent further damage.

- *Audiovisual and computer software.* Expensive and frequently used.

Circulation Systems and Procedures

Circulation Systems. Circulation systems vary according to the size and sophistication of the library. At a rudimentary level, a simple book card may be put into a pocket in each book or bound and unbound journal (if circulated). When the publication is borrowed, the card is taken out, the name of the borrower is added, and the date due is stamped on the card. Cards may be filed under due dates, author's name, or call number.

A nursing school library may use a circulation system such as the computer software program designed by Professional Software.

The Circulation Manager component of this system can be used without an online catalog. It provides a record of all items currently in circulation and a library client file. The program can print reports, overdue notices, overdue lists, labels, statistics, and form letters. Book cards are signed by the borrower and are filed manually by the librarian, to serve as evidence when users claim they do not have the item.

Other circulation procedures include the following actions:

- Notification of nursing staff offices when nurses are delinquent in returning library materials; notification of human resources when employees do not return library materials.
- Listing a phone number when a borrower is unaffiliated with the school, but works in the institution; full contact information—address and phone number—when the client is an outsider.
- Entry of books by call number, author, and title. Entry of journals are entered by title, volume, issue, and date; audiovisuals by format (slide, etc.), title, and call number.

If the nursing collection is part of a larger library or library system, its circulation and cataloging functions will probably be automated. An automated catalog, with many access points, can identify books and journals and tell the client whether a volume is available or charged out. It will also maintain an automated record of clients in which each registered borrower is bar-coded: When a transaction such as a loan occurs, the bar code is paired with the book, also bar-coded, and a record is created. If remote access to the automated catalog and networked databases is provided, the information they contain will be available from outside the library 24 hours a day.

Returns may be in the form of a book drop located in the library during hours of operation, and outside the library when the library is closed. In many institutions, material may also be returned via interdepartmental delivery.

COLLECTION MAINTENANCE

Arrangement of the Collection

Books in nursing collections may be shelved according to the National Library of Medicine Classification, preferably on open shelves or in open stack areas. Some libraries maintain a New Book Shelf on which newly cataloged books are displayed for a short time.

The simplest way to shelve journals is alphabetically by title. In the nursing library, they are usually retained for a minimum of 10 years, with the exception of core journals, such as the *American Journal of Nursing, RN, Nursing, Nursing Research,* and *Nursing Outlook,* which are kept longer. Depending upon the budget, two copies of the core titles are purchased; one is bound at the end of the year and placed in the rear of the library, until space is filled, at which time they are moved to a special storage area. Unbound journals may be shelved either with or separately from bound volumes. Another option is to display unbound journals on open shelves. In a typical nursing school library, current journals are displayed alphabetically by title on slant shelving with internal storage capacity for one year. Two, three, sometimes four journals occupy a position on each shelf. Allowance for bimonthly or weekly journals must be made since they will occupy more shelf space; as the first new issues of a year are received, the previous year's journals are placed with older issues in another area. Books and journals should be reshelved daily.

Current recreational magazines, hospital newsletters, and peripheral nursing materials (*AHA News, Nursing Spectrum,* student and hospital publications, etc.) are kept in a special display rack.

Lists of new books purchased are compiled by author and title and placed on student and faculty bulletin boards. When a book is a reference for students in a current course, it is placed on reserve to enable in-library access only to the entire class. If the book is of special interest to an instructor, the instructor is notified when it arrives and given the opportunity to borrow it before it is placed in general circulation.

122

COLLECTION CONTROL

Inventories and Weeding

Inventories. Inventories must be taken periodically, at least every two years, and at a time most convenient for users; that is, when it will not interfere with their work or study. Often, inventories are conducted in the summer when school is not in session, or during holidays, spring break, or other slow periods.

An inventory is an accounting of every item in the collection. The process begins by "reading the shelves" to be sure the collection is in alphanumeric order, and proceeds by comparing each item on the shelf with the official record, the shelflist or a printout from the online catalog. Missing items should be checked against circulation cards and flagged. Subject areas and titles should be noted for possible replacement, and unless the items are replaced, records should be withdrawn.

Records should be compiled to compare results with those of prior inventories, noting the number of losses, subject areas affected, cost of replacements. If necessary, these can then be used as proof to the administration of the urgency of securing the collection to prevent further losses.

Weeding. Weeding, too, must be done periodically and systematically. It is necessary to withdraw and discard materials that are out of date, out of scope, lacking in relevancy, superseded by new editions, in poor condition, or unused. Multiple copies can be discarded when shelves are crowded and use has become infrequent. Space requirements may also dictate withdrawals, particularly of older materials. The library's current collection policy should be used as a guide, but the faculty must be included in the final decision. "Classical" and historical publications usually are kept longer; but if it becomes necessary to discard them, they should be offered to archives rather than libraries with historical collections.

The librarian makes the decision to deselect, sometimes with the help of a faculty member as subject specialist. When discarding, the librarian pulls the book from the shelf, removes the book pocket and date due cards, and stamps the book "discarded" or "weeded." The shelflist card is pulled from the catalog, followed by subject, author, title cards, and tracings. A list of discards by call number should be kept to serve as a guide for assessing subject coverage. Discarded books then may be sold or donated to foreign medical schools, which often supplement their collections with such texts.

Securing the Library.   The library must take certain precautions to protect resources and users. As a deterrent to theft and entry of potentially troublesome individuals, there should be one main entrance and exit within sight of the library staff. Access policies should specify who may enter the library and what constitutes unacceptable behavior for library users. Such a written policy will serve as a basis for the librarian to evict a user whose access is prohibited or whose behavior is not acceptable.

All library personnel and users should be warned not to leave purses and other valuables unattended. If cash is collected, it should be kept in a safe or other secure location. Procedures for closing the library should be clearly posted so that the library can be secured in a timely fashion. Additional information on security is included in Chapter 2.

Theft, Loss, and Mutilation.   If the unauthorized removal of materials is a problem, an electronic theft detection system should be considered. Such a system alerts both the librarian as well as the user that unauthorized material is leaving the library; it can also serve as a powerful detection and deterrent tool. Cost analysis can justify the implementation of such a system if statistics are maintained that prove several years of heavy losses.

There are two kinds of electronic theft detection systems: a bypass system in which sensitized materials are passed around the sensing unit at checkout; and a system in which material is desensitized when it is checked out and resensitized when returned. In either case, a buzzer sounds at the library exit when materials are attempted to be taken out without clearing checkout. Some detection systems are integrated with automated circulation systems.

Mutilation of materials can be minimized by making photo-copiers readily available and by allowing materials to be checked out for photocopying in other areas. Pages removed by patrons can be replaced with photocopied pages.

INTERLIBRARY LOAN SERVICES

Policies

Interlibrary loan services enable libraries to provide materials they do not currently have on hand for their clients by borrowing them from other libraries. Interlibrary loan (ILL) policies vary from library to library, but in all cases, they should be in written form so that users can be aware of the procedures and so that the library can be consistent in providing services. Libraries cooperating in interlibrary loan services will have both borrowing and lending policies; therefore, knowledge of other library policies is useful when directing interlibrary loan requests. Interlibrary loans are governed by regulations of individual lending libraries, the "National Interlibrary Loan Code" (American Library Association, RASD, 1994b), the Copyright Act, and network agreements.

Borrowing Policies. Borrowing policies should state which users are eligible for interlibrary loan services, when it is appropri-ate to borrow materials, and the types of materials that may or may not be requested. Further, they should state the transmission means ordinarily used, the expected time of receipt of materials, and any fees that may be incurred. If another nearby library—hos-pital, academic, or public—has the material in question and is open to the nursing library's users, the nursing library may direct its users to that library rather than borrow for them.

Each library sets up its own restrictions on what it will loan. For example, some libraries will loan older materials and others will not.

Lending Policies. Lending policies should specify those li-braries eligible to borrow; indicate loan periods; and clearly state routine and expedited charges, renewal protocol, and the method for delivery and return of materials. The policy should also indicate the types of materials available and restricted.

Policies vary in regard to faxing articles. Most health sciences libraries will fax articles in medical emergencies, but will not routinely do so; instead they will use the mail or a delivery service in most cases. Those libraries that do fax usually charge additional fees. The Reference and Adult Services Division, ALA (American Library Association, RASD, 1994a), has issued guidelines and procedures for electronic delivery and telefacsimile in interlibrary loan.

Most libraries absorb the cost of interlibrary loans for their primary users, and do not charge, except for unusually expensive items; a few do charge fees to recover costs. However, users should be made aware that interlibrary lending does incur costs, and unless reciprocity exists, as among consortium members, libraries should expect to pay for interlibrary loans costs of staff time for processing, supplies, mailing, and other delivery charges. The most common rate paid by libraries is that established by the National Network of Libraries of Medicine (NN/LM), discussed in Chapter 10.

Procedures

Initiation of Requests by Patron. Patrons requesting interlibrary loans are usually asked to fill out interlibrary loan forms specific to the library. Such forms ask for information necessary to identify the requesting patron and determine his or her eligibility, and to locate the user when materials are received. They also ask for correct and complete information on the requested item. In a smaller library, where no forms are made available, the user may photocopy the reference as cited in an index and add his or her contact information.

Procedures for Borrowing Materials. Once the form is filled out completely and correctly by the patron, the nursing librarian will take the following steps:

1. Examine the form to be sure it is filled out correctly. Both the requester and the item to be borrowed must be adequately identified.

2. Confirm that the item requested is *not* in the library's collection.

3. Locate a library that owns the item. If it is nearby and accessible, send the user there in lieu of interlibrary borrowing.

4. Request the item electronically or by mailing a standard form. The American Library Association has designed a standard form available from most library supply houses.

5. Keep appropriate records so that the status of each request and the whereabouts of materials are known at all times.

6. When the item is received, contact the patron and deliver the item, indicating date to be returned and whether the item may be renewed. The exception is when the user is given a photocopy of an article, in which case, he or she may keep it.

7. When the item is returned by the patron, release the records and return the item immediately to the lending library.

8. If the item is not returned on the date due, recover it from the client and return it immediately to the lending library.

DOCLINE is the National Library of Medicine's automated system for locating and ordering articles. The librarian or clerk enters information into a computer, and DOCLINE subsequently inputs the information to SERLINE, the National Library of Medicine's online serials database, to find a library that owns the item, then initiates an interlibrary loan request for it. Because this system is automatic, it requires little experience of the person locating materials, although a knowledgeable librarian may choose to override the system's choice for a preferred supplier.

The Union Catalog of Medical Periodicals (UCMP), RLIN, and OCLC also serve as locating tools. The UCMP is available both on microfiche and online, and lists holdings of many libraries. It is incorporated into SERLINEonline, which, as just mentioned, serves as the locating tool for DOCLINE.

Both OCLC and RLIN are electronic databases, sometimes called bibliographic utilities, created by cooperative cataloging systems. Smaller libraries that do not use these systems for cataloging can access the data online. Some consortia, like the Medical Library Center of New York, sponsor group subscriptions to OCLC.

Library Staff Procedures for Lending Materials.   Upon receipt of a loan request from another library, the first step is to determine that library's eligibility to borrow. Then:

1. Determine whether the item is owned and available for loan or for photocopying.
2. Record the transaction. Charge the item out, if a book, and determine the date return is expected (loan period plus mailing time).
3. Send the item to the requesting library, indicating the date of return expected. Books are usually sent by United States mail or by a delivery service such as United Parcel Service.
4. Follow up on all items not returned by the due date and send reminders (overdue notices).
5. If the book or other item is not returned, bill the borrowing library for the cost of the book plus handling (recataloging, etc.).

Copyright Restrictions

Fair Use.   Making a single copy of a journal article for interlibrary loans, for research, and for other noncommercial uses is

128

usually acceptable under the principle of fair use. However, photocopy regulations make it illegal to copy whole issues of journals. In addition, the same title cannot be requested more than five times in one year; a journal used that frequently should be purchased, or royalty fees should be paid to the publisher. Consequently, the librarian should devise and maintain a system to record requests in order to track when "fair use" will be exceeded. The Medical Library Association has a useful booklet covering copyright restrictions (Medical Library Association, 1989). Additional information on copyright is included in Chapter 2.

Consortia and Commercial Document Delivery

Consortia. A group of libraries may set up a consortium for reciprocal provision of loans and may or may not offer other services. Fees and borrowing regulations are set up by member libraries. The Medical Library Center (MLC) of New York is such a consortium. The Union Catalog of Medical Periodicals is a product of MLC, which also offers a truck delivery service and storage space.

Borrowing and lending policies that apply to libraries with no specific agreements are fully described in the "National Interlibrary loan code for the United States, 1993" (American Library Association, RASD, 1994b), and *The Interlibrary Loan Practices Handbook* (Boucher, 1995).

The ILL policies, procedures, and practices of the National Network of Libraries of Medicine (NN/LM) affect all health sciences libraries and is discussed in Chapter 10. The various Regional Medical Libraries of the NN/LM will usually supply a regional interlibrary loan/document delivery policy manual upon request. See Chapter 10 for a list of the Regional Medical Libraries.

Nursing libraries may participate in regional consortia of health sciences libraries or in consortia that involve different kinds of libraries, such as academic, public, and special libraries. An example of a local network is the New Jersey Health Sciences Network, a free reciprocal interlibrary lending network that became operational in 1981. Requirements included an institutional membership in Health Sciences Library Association of New Jersey (HSLANJ). In 1986, this network expanded to include health science librarians in New York, New Jersey, and Pennsylvania. The Basic Health Sciences Libraries (BHSL) Network now operates in 10 states.

Commercial Document Delivery. The use of commercial suppliers such as University Microfilms Incorporated (UMI), Institute for Scientific Information's The Genuine Article (TGA), Carl's UnCover, Faxon Finder, The Information Store (TIF), and Information on Demand (IOD) are sometimes used to supplement, or as an alternative to, ILL services provided by in-house library staff. Some libraries choose to obtain photocopies of articles through commercial document delivery services rather than from other libraries. The price paid to the supplier includes a royalty paid to the publisher (Kurosman & Durniak, 1994). Costs incurred are usually higher than for interlibrary loans, and must be watched closely as few articles are obtained for the average costs estimated by the supplier, but may be offset by speed of access or reduced staff time (Mancini, 1996).

Libraries often use this route when materials are not readily available from other libraries. Many go directly to University Microfilms to obtain dissertations, because it is easier to order them in microform from one supplier than to contact individual schools, some of which do not lend.

In general, as libraries decrease expenses for journal subscriptions and book collections, they must realize that interlibrary loan costs will increase.

CONCLUSION

Changes in the health care delivery system and developments in technology draw a dynamic backdrop for the provision of information and educational services. Libraries will change as they adopt and adapt to new technologies and their users become more proficient information gatherers. Libraries will adopt new policies and procedures, and may look different, but their basic purpose, providing information and educational services, will remain.

REFERENCES

American Library Association, ACRL. (1990). Guidelines for extended campus library services. C&RL News, 51, 353–355.

American Library Association, RASD. (1994a). Guidelines and procedures for telefacsimile and electronic delivery of interlibrary loan requests and materials. Reference Quarterly, 34(1), 32–33.

American Library Association, RASD. (1994b). National Interlibrary Loan Code for the United States, 1993. Reference Quarterly, 33, 477–479.

American Library Association, RSTD Filing Committee. (1980). ALA Filing Rules. Chicago: American Library Association.

Blythe, J., Royle, J. A., Oolup, P., Potvin, C., & Smith, S. D. (1995). Linking the professional literature to nursing practice: challenges and opportunities. AAOHN Journal, 43(6), 342–345.

Boucher, V. (1995). Interlibrary loan practices handbook (2nd ed.). Chicago: American Library Association.

Brandon, A. N., & Hill, D. R. (1996). Selected list of nursing books and journals. Nursing Outlook, 44(1), 56–66.

Bunting, A. (1994). Legal considerations for document delivery services. Bulletin of the Medical Library Association, 82, 183–187.

Canavan, K. (1996). Nurses take the lead in consumer education. American Nurse, 28(1), 1, 8.

Cibbarelli, P. R., Gerrel, F. H., & Kratzert, M. (1993). Choosing among the options for patron access databases: Print, online, CD-ROM, or locally mounted. The Reference Librarian, (39), 85–97.

Cutter, C. A. (1969). Cutter-Sanborn three-figure author table (Swanson-Swift revision). Chicopee, MA: H. R. Huntting Co.

Interagency Council on Information Resources for Nursing. (1996). Essential nursing references. N&HC Perspectives on Community, 17, 255–259.

Kascus, M., & Aguilar, W. (1988). Providing library support to off-campus programs. College & Research Libraries, 49, 29–37.

Kurosman, K., & Durniak, B. A. (1994). Document delivery: A comparison of commercial document suppliers and interlibrary loan services. College & Research Libraries, 55(2), 129–139.

Lamont, J. (1996). Friendly CD ROMs from the federal government. Computers in Libraries, 16, 68–74.

Mancini, A. D. (1996). Evaluating commercial document suppliers: Improving access to current journal literature. College & Research Libraries, 57, 123–131.

McAfooes, J. (1995). An overview of hardware and software grants for nursing education. *Interactive Healthcare Newsletter, 11*(7/8), 2–3.

Medical Library Association. (1989). *The copyright law and the health sciences librarian* (Rev. ed.). Chicago: Medical Library Association.

Medial Library Association. (1996). The librarian's role in the provision of consumer health information and patient education. *Bulletin of the Medical Library Association, 84,* 238–239.

Mountainside Hospital School of Nursing. (1996–1997). *Guidebook* (pp. 23–24). Montclair, NJ: Mountainside Hospital School of Nursing. (Unpublished)

Mountainside Hospital School of Nursing. (1997). *Systemic plan of evaluation* (p. 15). Montclair, NJ: Mountainside Hospital School of Nursing. (Unpublished)

Mullaly-Quijas, P., Ward, D. H., & Woelfl, N. (1994). Using focus groups to discover health professionals' information needs: A regional marketing study. *Bulletin of the Medical Library Association, 82,* 305–311.

National Library of Medicine. (1995). *National library of medicine classification scheme for the shelf arrangement of materials in the medical field and its related sciences* (5th ed.). Bethesda, MD: National Library of Medicine.

Rees, A. M. (1994). *Consumer health information source book.* Phoenix, AZ: Oryx Press.

Schockley, J. S. (1988). *Information resources for nursing, a guide.* New York: National League for Nursing.

Silverstein, J. L. (1995). Strengthening the links between health sciences information users and providers. *Bulletin of the Medical Library Association, 83,* 407–417.

Simmons, H. L. (1991). Accreditation expectations for library support of off-campus programs. *Library Trends, 39,* 388–404.

Spath, M., & Buttlar, L. (1996). Brief communications. Information and research needs of acute-care clinical nurses. *Bulletin of the Medical Library Association, 84,* 112–116.

Strauch, K., Linton, R., & Cohen, C. (1992). *Library research guide to nursing: Illustrated search strategy & sources.* Ann Arbor, MI: Pierian Press.

Taylor, R. S. (1968). Question-negotiation and information-seeking in libraries. *College & Research Libraries, 29*(3), 178–194.

Tyler, J. K., & Switzer, J. H. (1991). Meeting the information needs of nursing students: A library instruction module for a nursing research class. *Medical Reference Services Quarterly, 10*(3), 39–44.

Wehmeyer, J. M. (1995). MDX Health Digest: A consumer health database. *Medical Reference Services Quarterly, 14*(2), 53–60.

Wood, E. H. (1995). Legi-Slate: A federal information database. *Medical Reference Services Quarterly, 14*(4), 1–10.

Woods, S. E. (1996). Combined health information database. *Medical References Services Quarterly, 15*(2), 53–59.

RESOURCE REFERENCES*

Allergi, F. (Ed.). (1995). *Educational services in health sciences libraries*. Metuchen, NJ: Medical Library Association and Scarecrow Press.

Buchanan, H. S., & Marshall, J. G. (1995). Benchmarking reference services: Step-by-step. *Medical Reference Services Quarterly, 14*(3), 1–13.

Clamp, G. L., Ballard, M. P., & Gough, S. (1994). *Sources for nursing research*. London: Library Association Publishing.

Gale Directory of Databases. (1996). In M. Alampi (Ed.) and K. L. Miller, & P. Lewon (Assoc. Eds.). *Vol 1: Online databases; Vol 2: CD-ROM, diskette, magnetic tape, handheld, and batch access database products*. Detroit, MI: Gale Research.

Guide to Reference Books. (1996). R. Balay (Ed.). (11th ed.). Chicago: American Library Association.

Interagency Council on Information Resources for Nursing. (1996). Essential nursing references. *N&HC Perspectives on Community, 17*, 255–259.

Lamont, J. (1996). Friendly CD-ROMs from the federal government. *Computers in Libraries, 16*, 68–74.

Lipscomb, C. E. (Ed.). (1996). *Information access and delivery in health sciences libraries*. Metuchen, NJ: Medical Library Association and Scarecrow Press.

Marshall, J. G., & Buchanan, H. S. (1995). Benchmarking reference services: An introduction. *Medical Reference Services Quarterly, 14*(3), 59–73.

Matthews, M., & Brennan, P. (Eds.). (1995). *Copyright, public policy, and the scholarly community*. Washington, DC: Association of Research Libraries.

Payson, E. (1995). The vertical file: Retain or discard? *College & Research Libraries, 56*, 123–132.

Rees, A. M. (1994). *Consumer health information source book*. Phoenix, AZ: Oryx Press.

Rees, A. M. (Ed.). (1991). *Managing consumer health information services*. Phoenix, AZ: Oryx Press.

Roper, F. W., & Boorkman, J. A. (1994). *Introduction to reference sources in the health sciences* (3rd ed.). Chicago, IL: Medical Library Association; Metuchen, NJ: Scarecrow Press.

Walford, A. J. (1989). *Walford's guide to reference materials: Vol. 1, science and technology*. London: Library Association.

Wood, M. S. (Ed.). (1994). *Reference and information services in health sciences libraries*. Metuchen, NJ: Medical Library Association and Scarecrow Press.

---

* Many of the publications on this list are available in public libraries or in libraries that are members of the NN/LM, which is discussed in Chapter 10. Additional resources are included at the end of Chapter 5.

SUGGESTED READINGS

Bair, A. H., Brown, L. P., Pugh, L. C., & Borucki, L. C. (1996). Taking the bite out of CRISP: Strategies on using and conducting searches in the Computer Retrieval of Information on Scientific Projects Database. *Computers in Nursing, 14,* 218–224.

Bell, S. J. (1993). Providing remote access to CD-ROMS: Some practical advice. *CD-ROM Professional, 6*(1), 43–47.

Burnham, J. F. (1994). Information management education for students in the health care professions: A coordinated, integrated plan. *Medical Reference Services Quarterly, 13,* 45–62.

Cibbarelli, P. R., Gertel, E. H., & Kratzert, M. (1993). Choosing among the options for patron access databases: Print, online, CD-ROM, or locally mounted. *The Reference Librarian,* (39), 85–97.

Davis, T. L. (1993). Acquisition of CD-ROM databases for local area networks. *The Journal of Academic Librarianship, 19*(2), 68–71.

Delozier, E. P. (1996). Internet access and connectivity: An explanation. *Medical Reference Services Quarterly, 15*(1), 63–69.

George, L. A. (1993). Fee-based information services and document delivery. *Wilson Library Bulletin, 67*(6), 41–44, 112.

Greenfield, L., Tellman, J., & Brin, B. (1996). A model for teaching the Internet: Preparation and practice. *Computers in Libraries, 16*(3), 22–25.

Hankel, M. L., & Skiffington, F. W. (1991). Accessibility and reference use of the depository collection in college and university libraries. *The Reference Librarian,* (32), 71–84.

Harter, S. P., & Kim, H. J. (1996). Accessing electronic journals and other E-publications: An empirical study. *College & Research Libraries, 57,* 440–455.

Hernon, P., & Heisser, D. C. (1991). GPO regional depositories. *The Reference Librarian,* (32), 43–55.

Kroll, H. R. (1990). The responsive reference collection: Planning for service versus self-service in the reference area. *The Reference Librarian,* (29), 9–19.

Lessin, B. M. (1991). Library models for the delivery of support services to off-campus academic programs. *Library Trends, 39,* 405–423.

Lynden, F. C. (1994). Remote access issues: Pros and cons. *Journal of Library Administration, 20*(1), 19–36.

Mancini, A. D. (1996). Evaluating commercial document suppliers: Improving access to current journal literature. *College and Research Libraries, 57,* 123–131.

Mathews, E., & Tyckoson, D. A. (1990). A program for the systematic weeding of the reference collection. *Reference Librarian,* (29), 129–143.

Nolan, C. W. (1993). The confidentiality of interlibrary loan records. *The Journal of Academic Librarianship, 19*(2), 81–86.

Reed, M. H. (1987). *The copyright primer for librarians and educators.* Chicago: American Library Association; Washington, DC: National Education Association.

Stanley, N. M. (1995). Purchasing electronic resources: An acquisitions perspective. *The Acquisitions Librarian,* (13/14), 153–163.

Van Goethem, J. (1995). Buying, leasing, and connecting to electronic information: The changing scene of library acquisitions. *The Acquisitions Librarian,* (13/14), 165–174.

APPENDIX
SUGGESTED INFORMATION FOR A
REFERENCE POLICY STATEMENT
(MOUNTAINSIDE HOSPITAL SCHOOL
OF NURSING, 1996–1997, PP. 23–24)

1. Who formulates the policy? Is it reviewed and revised regularly?
2. What are the library's objectives?
   a. To provide appropriate information related to nursing.
   b. To promote independent use of the library's resources.
3. What types of services are offered?
   a. Answers to direct questions.
   b. Assistance in using the catalog systems and various indexes (manual and online).
   c. Locating resources.
   d. Orientation and library instruction.
   e. Searching online indexes for answers to specific questions.
   f. Searching subjects for course bibliographies.
4. Who are the primary clientele?
   a. Students enrolled at the School of Nursing.
   b. Faculty.
   c. Students in related programs.
   d. Employees and staff of the school and the hospital.
   e. Others: Community and students enrolled at other colleges; referrals made by public libraries, school libraries, law firms, corporations seeking health-related information, who may use the library, but may not borrow.
5. Hours?
   a. Evening and weekend hours the library is open, if any.
   b. Hours when student monitors or volunteers keep the library open.
   c. Hours the librarian is available (staffing).
   d. Must outsiders make appointments before coming?
6. Use of Equipment
   a. Is there a charge for photocopying? Faxing? Literature searching? Interlibrary loan?
   b. Is a microfilm/microfiche reader/printer available? Is there a charge? Per page? Per article?
   c. Are typewriters or computers available?
   d. Is there access to computers for online searching and access to the Internet?
   e. Are audiovisual aids available?

5

Collection Development and Evaluation

Jonathan DeForest Eldredge, MLS, PhD

Collection development provides coherence and establishes priorities in an environment where demands for information resources far exceed budgetary constraints. The need for reliable and timely health sciences information most likely will increase in the foreseeable future. The Joint Commission on Accreditation of Healthcare Associations (JCAHO) in recent years has emphasized the need for information provided by health sciences libraries (1996). Studies that link improved patient care and cost containment to the current health sciences literature (Marshall, 1992) have caught the attention of health policy experts and decision makers (McClure, 1995) which can only increase demands upon library collections.

This chapter addresses issues relating to collection development and evaluation that may be applicable to large or small collections of nursing resources.

Needs Assessment

Nursing collections are intended to provide reliable and primarily current information resources to primary clientele. These collections may serve any of the following purposes, depending upon

Jonathan DeForest Eldredge

the parent institution's mission: clinical care, research, education, and accreditation. The priority attached to any of these should define the goals and objectives of a collection development program. A health sciences center library probably will serve all four purposes, whereas an undergraduate academic library serving a nursing degree program will focus primarily upon the educational purpose, with some attention paid to accreditation purposes. A hospital library collection, a departmental library, nursing center library, or even a small collection at a nurses' station will, by contrast, concentrate primarily upon clinical care.

Nurses approach information from a highly *multidisciplinary* perspective. Practicing nurses in specialties tend to delve into comparable medical specialties or associated allied health literatures to find information needed for their practices. Nursing students and faculty members frequently consult the literatures of the social sciences, behavioral sciences, and biological sciences as well as medicine to conduct their research.

The information needs of practicing nurses tend to be closely tied to their clinical environments. Small collections found at nurses' stations often include pharmacology sources, handbooks, and texts from parallel medical specialties. A cardiac unit, for example, might contain a leading cardiology textbook. Delman (1982) notes that one should not infer too much from the types or volume of clinical patient care in a hospital environment when determining actual information needs. As he observes, ". . . only a small portion of a hospital's clinical problems are actually significant information problems" (p. 405). Still, Colglazier (1996) has found that the clinical orientation of these information needs generally have a causal relationship with collection use.

Needs assessment efforts permeate many aspects of collection development, even those to promote use of collections. The book and journal selection process can include making contact with requesters when titles are suggested for purchase not only to notify them about the decision, but to solicit their views about the collection. Once requested books arrive, the requester and any other potentially interested clientele can be notified. Such simple promotional measures normally are met with noteworthy appreciation. Similarly, notifying potentially interested clientele when the

138

library begins subscribing to a journal builds obvious clientele satisfaction with collections. Likewise, clientele appreciate the opportunity to at least comment upon proposed cancelations. Subject lists of current nursing journal subscriptions are frequently employed to promote use of a nursing collection to faculty, students, and affiliated clinical nurses. In the needs assessment process, understanding client interests will greatly aid in promoting collections. Therefore, any means that can be found to communicate how collections will meet the needs of clientele should be seriously considered.

COLLECTION DEVELOPMENT POLICIES

Once an assessment has determined that a library (or at least a collection) will serve identifiable needs, some sort of policy statement that defines the purpose of the collection is a reasonable next step. Collection development policies vary in complexity and detail, ranging in length from less than one page to about 100 pages.

Carpenter (1984) states that collection development policies may serve as planning documents, communication tools, and foundations for resource sharing with other libraries. "Without these a library is engaged only in acquiring—spending money and adding books—not in rationally and systematically developing its collection." He adds, "Writing a policy compels the librarian to develop a rationale, a plan for acquiring materials—to ask, 'What is the library acquiring, and why?'" (pp. 43–44). The collection development policy links the library's activities to the mission of the parent institution. It also outlines the selection directions taken by the library so that these rationales can be communicated to customers, or to other librarians at other institutions who may not want to duplicate information available at a particular library.

Controversy surrounds the subject of collection development policies. Cargill (1984) argues against them since these time-consuming projects tend to foster inflexibility as institutional priorities or clientele change. Snow (1996) has presented one of the most articulate critiques of collection development policies, which echoes many of Cargill's misgivings. Should a library invest in the

139

creation of a policy, he asks, when it needs to be updated "almost continuously to reflect changes" (p. 193).

The real argument in the debate seems to revolve around the amount of detail necessary to incorporate in a collection development policy. All involved seem to agree that at least a brief collection development policy document that relates the parent institution's mission to the purposes of the collection is useful, and should include statements about which subjects to include in the collection. Statements about the subject scope should also indicate the level of coverage. For example, White (1995) outlines the Research Libraries Group (RLG) levels of coverage for subjects as minimal, basic, instructional support, research, and comprehensive (p. 5). In this regard, broad policy statements may suffice, if given the flexibility to undergo revisions to reflect changing goals and needs of clientele. Then, if the library needs to integrate greater detail into the basic document, it still may do so to account for inevitable changes and exceptions.

JOURNALS SELECTION

The ratio of journals to other media such as books or CD-ROMs in a nursing collection will vary dramatically according to the initial needs assessment. Burdick, Butler, and Sullivan (1993) suggest that an 88-to-12 ratio of journals to books profile would be appropriate, based upon the reliance of each medium found through their citation analyses. However, the research orientation of this study and the assumptions made by the investigators need to be taken in account when considering this proposed ratio. Other collections may need to pursue a different ratio suited for clients' needs. A nursing station or a departmental library in a teaching hospital, for example, may require an inverse ratio of books to journals.

Purposes of Journals

Health sciences journals provide the means for rapid communication of research results, clinical experiences, ideas, and information.

Journals frequently comply with quality control standards (e.g., editorial boards, peer review) to increase the likelihood that, whenever possible, empirical methods have been appropriately employed to report information. Most journals are published according to established schedules, usually at weekly, biweekly, monthly, bimonthly, quarterly, or semiannual intervals, and most include articles that focus upon narrowly defined topics. Although journals still are published predominantly in print, increasingly, they are produced in other formats, including audio- and videocassette, CD-ROM, diskette, and in online versions.

Technically speaking, journals belong to a broader class of regularly produced publications known as serials, which include annual reviews, conference proceedings, and newsletters. But because most serials in health sciences collections consist of journals, the following discussion can apply to these other types of serials under the more specific term of journals.

The now famous Rochester Study (Marshall, 1992) conducted in upstate New York evaluated results gained from practitioners who had sought answers to their clinical questions in journal articles. Of all participants, 80 percent stated that they probably or definitely handled an aspect of patient care differently due to what they learned from journal literature. Specific behavior changes consisted of: diagnosis 29 percent, choice of tests 51 percent, choice of drugs 45 percent, reduced length of stay 19 percent, and advice given to the patient 72 percent (p. 169). These impressive results have caught the interest of policymakers in Washington as they grapple with current trends in health care (McClure, 1995). Although the specific implications of these studies to nursing practice have not yet been determined, the importance of one's professional and continuing education via the journal literature as discussed by Weaver (1993) suggests that these studies are highly relevant. Complementary studies (with nurses' use of the journal literature reported by Blythe & Royle, 1993 or journals use by more broadly defined health care practitioner groups as reported by Delman, 1982 and Colglazier, 1996) point to greater importance attached to using the journal literature by nurses in the future.

Jonathan DeForest Eldredge

Predicting Potential Use of a Journal

Relevance to Clientele. The multidisciplinary orientation of the nursing profession requires the collection development librarian to consider a wide variety of possible subscriptions to serve potential clientele. Nurses' interests can parallel specialties in medicine, the biological sciences, social sciences, behavioral sciences, and management subjects.

To subscribe to a journal implies a long-term commitment to the collection and the organization it serves. In particular, it involves a long-term commitment to continue buying the subscription for at least three to five years due to customer expectations based upon their observed behavior in using collections. Unfortunately, journal subscriptions in the health sciences generally are expensive and prone to dramatic inflationary increases, which often bewilders librarians. Lewis (1989) describes the journals market as a natural monopoly because journal publishing, as we know it, cannot occur without subsidization. Library budgets are one source for this subsidization even though these budgets have diminished in relation to parent institutions' overall finances in recent years (Henderson, 1995). Health sciences journals have an elite readership, hence are not produced in large quantities and cannot offset costs through advertisements. These factors tend to make health sciences journals expensive in contrast to popular magazines such as *Time* or *Newsweek*.

Any discussion of relevance surrounding the decision to subscribe to a journal must define "relevance" in terms of a sustained interest over several years. What will library clientele want to read month after month, year after year? Many journals have high appeal for brief periods of a year or less, then are canceled due to lack of perceived relevance to clients at a later date, signaling a poor investment for the organization. During this short period, scarce resources will have been devoted to paying for the subscription at the higher institutional rate and tracking its receipt and usage; and the journal will have been occupying limited space on shelves.

One informal method for determining the relevance of a title is to simply ask library clientele who have suggested that the collection include a specific title why they think it would be an important investment. Sometimes a journal title—for example, a highly specialized one on quality assurance—will be recommended for purchase due to a client's lack of knowledge of what the collection contains; that is, he or she may not realize that many journals already in the collection contain more relevant articles on, in this case, quality assurance. This probably indicates a need to better promote the collection to potential clients.

On the other hand, a request for a new journal may alert the librarian to an emerging program, a new clinic, or previously underrepresented patient population. Collections intended to serve clinical programs need to reflect the major patient populations frequenting those clinical areas. A review of the Diagnostic Related Groups (DRGs) and total drug costs for the clinical areas served can provide a reality check on the subjects that should be represented in the collection (Colglazier, 1996). Although Delman (1982) cautions that ". . . not every frequently occurring and significant clinical problem represents a significant information problem" (p. 401). A review of the staffing and patient care loads for existing nursing stations or large medical departments (Pediatrics, Oncology, etc.) may lend insight into the major clinical emphases of an institution. If the collection serves an academic program, a careful review of existing courses, areas of concentration, and graduate degrees should direct the subjects represented by journals subscriptions. Major research areas of the institution, if any, also need to be reflected.

Interlibrary Loan Use.   Examining the aggregate use of frequently requested journals via interlibrary loan represents one of the most popular methods for identifying possible new subscriptions for libraries, since it seems reasonable to subscribe to an unowned journal in the presence of such obvious demand by customers. Nevertheless, there are many pitfalls associated with this indicator of potential use if it is not analyzed thoroughly.

Interlibrary loan records need to be checked carefully to determine first whether heavy demand for a certain journal recurs year after year. A sharp upward demand spike for only one year may represent a dramatic interest connected with a short-term project conducted by an individual or a small group of researchers. For example, a small group may have been writing a research grant proposal or conducting specialized research during that year, which generated heavy demand for a specific title through interlibrary loan. A unique patient problem or a minor epidemic in the clinical setting also may generate sudden surges in demand that will not continue in subsequent years.

When interlibrary loan demand persists for more than one year, the question that must be answered is, can it be attributed only to an individual's solitary albeit sustained interest over time? The subsequent question in such a case is: Will anyone other than this individual ever want this title? The answers to these questions must factor in the perceived value of this individual or group to the institution. You may want to subscribe to this journal if, for instance, this individual or a small team of investigators attracts 1,000 patients per year or secures a few million dollars in research funding for the institution each year. Of course, such individuals may have the resources, and the advantages, of subscribing to the journal at lower individual rates.

When many different clients representing diverse departments within the parent organization request unique articles from the same journal title via interlibrary loan, it becomes probable that subscribing to the popular title will be a solid investment for the institution, especially if those who have requested these articles are satisfied with the quality of the articles from the unowned journal. Still, several more critical tests of the heavy demand indicator need to be applied before ordering the subscription. One must ask: Are most articles requested from a special issue on a perennially popular subject? Are most requests for the same landmark or classic articles? Lacroix (1994) has found that fewer than 1 percent of all interlibrary loans per year exceed 10 requests for the same article, so this phenomenon of recurring requests for the same articles may be relatively isolated. Lacroix also discovered that of the 4 million requests examined, about 19,000 requests per year (p. 364) were for unique journal titles. In addition, citations on requests for a certain journal title that date back five or more years may indicate that the journal may have published salient results at one time, but has declined in both relevance and quality during recent years. Journals are ever-changing human institutions that operate under different editors, editorial boards, organizations, and publishers over the period of a decade. These variances can affect the quality of the journal.

The cost of journal ownership goes beyond the subscription price to include: organizing its place in the collection for efficient access; determining shelf space requirements and any use studies; and maintaining desirable environmental conditions to preserve these publications. When compared to the costs of access via interlibrary loan, the collection development librarian may elect to continue obtaining the articles from other libraries. Interlibrary loan requests at the cost of about $20 per request (Roche, 1993) may be more economical than subscribing to the actual journal. Thus, the collection development librarian needs to factor the total anticipated need for the journal on site. For example, certain clinical journals prone to urgent requests may be better candidates for purchase even if the costs of on-site access slightly exceed the cost of obtaining them via interlibrary loan. In recent years, the analysis of costs associated with access versus ownership of a journal subscription has been complicated by rising copyright fees (Bruwelheide, 1995) connected with obtaining a photocopy of an article.

Larger metropolitan areas may be home to other libraries with subscriptions to journals in demand by your clientele, precluding the need in your collection, provided demand for interlibrary loans is not too great and price is not too high. Common sense is often a reliable guide to these decisions: If library clientele are clamoring for the purchase of popular and inexpensive journals such as *American Journal of Nursing* or *Nursing*, it would be wise to subscribe even if another library five miles away owns these same titles.

Index Coverage.   Whether an indexing service covers the contents of a journal will many times determine if a library elects to subscribe to that journal. Most journals' use can be attributed to library clientele generating citations to articles on subjects of interest through either print or electronic indexing services. This access via indexing coverage greatly increases the possibility that journals will be used, an important ingredient in gaining a return on the investment of subscription costs. Many of the journals of interest to nurses are indexed in the *RNdex Top 100,* the *Cumulative Index to Nursing & Allied Health Literature* (CINAHL), the *International Nursing Index* (INI), *Index Medicus,* or MEDLINE. Both the INI and CINAHL provide a list of journals indexed in each quarterly issue and annual cumulation. CINAHL also includes the addresses of the publishers of all the journals indexed. Journals indexed in *Index Medicus* are included in the printed *List of Journals Indexed in Index Medicus, 1996.* Journals indexed in MEDLINE, AIDSLINE, and HealthSTAR are included in the *List of Serials Indexed for Online Users, 1996.*

For some types of journals, access to contents via indexing services will be far less important. Current awareness journals that either summarize or refer to articles in other journals serve functions similar to indexes. Review journals that devote their quarterly or bimonthly volumes to central themes might be another exception. These titles in the "clinics" or "seminars" genre such as *Nursing Clinics of North America* can be helpful additions to your collection as long as efforts are made to catalog them on a volume-by-volume basis, or through some other mode of easy access to their contents. Journals that report largely news may be another exception, although newsletters normally fulfill this news-reporting function. The general rule of thumb in making exceptions is to ensure that library clientele have alternative modes of access to these types of publications.

Quality Filter Guidelines

Once the relevancy of the subject matter of a journal has been determined, it can be evaluated according to certain quality standards, which can be done by implementing a number of basic techniques. Although some of these techniques require time to apply, they are essential if the journal collection is to reflect high standards of quality.

Expert Evaluation by Library Clientele. Nurses or other health care professionals affiliated with the parent institution who

146

represent a variety of health care specialties may be able to share their expertise by evaluating a journal under consideration. Sample issues can often be obtained from the publisher or the serials vendor servicing the library, although frequently a second or third follow-up request by the librarian might be necessary to secure them. (Experts find it much easier to evaluate the actual sample issues of a journal rather than just a printout of citations and abstracts of articles published by the journal that can be generated by an online literature search.) Clinically oriented evaluators may find the inventory of key characteristics of a journal developed by Sievert, McKinin, Johnson, Reid, and Mitchell (1996, p. 354) to be helpful.

The one pitfall of using experts to evaluate journals stems from a natural enthusiasm they will have for the subject matter of the journal under consideration. They may rate the journal with high marks in the hope that their subject interests will be more strongly represented in the collection through a decision to subscribe to the journal in question. This pitfall can be minimized by asking experts to compare the potential subscription with an actual subscription already in your collection. Ask if they would cancel the existing subscription in their area in favor of buying the potential subscription. Setting up the evaluation as an either-or choice may provide you with a realistic and critical evaluation of all titles in an expert's subject area, especially the journal under consideration. A modified sample evaluation form used for this purpose at the University of New Mexico Health Sciences Center Library is in Appendix B.

Peer Review. Health sciences journals vary widely in the manner by which they select manuscripts and prepare them for publication. Peer review (Burnham, 1990) involves a journal editor distributing submitted manuscripts to at least one expert in the field for critical evaluation. Positive evaluations of manuscripts by these experts usually leads to eventual publication of the manuscript in the journal.

The collection development librarian needs to consider the relevance and importance of peer review to the library's clientele when selecting new journal subscriptions. Although controversy surrounds the practices of peer review, most librarians consider peer-reviewed journals to be higher-quality publications when weighing criteria for journals selection.

Journal Reviews. Journal reviews in *JAMA: Journal of the American Medical Association* often have relevance to nurses even though the target audiences for these reviews are clinical physicians and medical librarians (Eakin, 1993). These rigorous reviews of new journals of potential relevance for a nursing collection usually appear in the first issue for each month. A master list of reviews published for the years 1992–1996, has been compiled (Eldredge, 1997).

Brandon-Hill Lists of Journals. The first selective list of nursing journals published by Alfred Brandon and Dorothy Hill (1979) contained 45 journals and 2 indexing services. Five journal titles from the original 1979 list are still in publication, but no longer appear on the 1994 list. A few journals have changed titles over the years. Thus, the original list has remained fairly constant. Subsequent lists have been expanded, though, to add more journals. The 1994 Brandon-Hill list contains 77 nursing journals.

The Brandon-Hill nursing list and its counterpart for small medical libraries should not be mistakenly viewed as a "standard collection" of journals. Unfortunately, various accrediting organizations have placed an inappropriate emphasis upon libraries owning titles that appear on these lists. This "cookbook" approach to developing collections should be avoided at all costs. A library should be tailored to the needs of its primary clientele. Brandon and Hill themselves admonish their readers to consider local circumstances and to exercise professional judgment when they write: "We intend and have always intended that our list should be used only as a guideline for making one aware of the current literature that we would select for a nursing collection . . ." (1994, p. 71). Nevertheless, the Brandon-Hill list of journals offers collection development librarians a starting point for identifying possible subscriptions. These journals, regardless of their relevance to local customer interests tend to exhibit high quality. By employing the other criteria described in this chapter in conjunction with the

Brandon-Hill lists, librarians can select quality journals for their collection.

Reputation of the Publisher. Only by informal, off-the-record conversations with librarians does the importance of a publisher's reputation become apparent in the process of journal selection. Some of the principal complaints about publishers are their price-gouging practices through highly inflationary annual subscription price increases, poor-quality articles, the tendency to market faddish subject areas, not supplying requested sample issues for review, and not publishing on schedule.

Cohn, Brondoli, and Bedell (1996) offer some insight into the more positive, value-added contributions by publishers to create a high-quality journal. As a general rule, when a reputable professional association either publishes or oversees the commercial publication of a journal, librarians tend to view it as a higher quality title.

Reputation of Editors and Editorial Board Members. When experts evaluate potential journal subscriptions, part of the process should include evaluations of the editors' and editorial board members' reputations. The collection development librarian can otherwise review these individuals' publications and conduct citation analyses on these publications.

Citation Analysis. One measure of a journal's quality might be the number of times within a recent time frame, such as the past three years, that authors have cited a particular journal (Garfield, 1996). Citation analysis, normally employed to determine an author's possible significance in a field, also may be used to measure the significance of a journal within a discipline (Garfield, 1972). Unfortunately, the sheer number of articles published by a journal within a given year can distort the significance ranking of the journal unless methodologically corrected (Rousseau & Van Hooydonk, 1996). In general, citation analysis methods have an array of limitations (Schoch, 1994, p. 35). Furthermore, as one moves into the subjects of clinical medicine and the nursing profession, the

Journal Citation Reports have greatly diminished utility for determining journal quality since clinically oriented health sciences journals are barely within scope for these reports.

Price and Price Inflation History. The collection development librarian has the difficult talk of allocating scarce financial resources to meet customer demands in the most cost-effective manner. The price of a journal must be factored into any analysis of its quality. Two preliminary questions must be asked by the journal selector: Will predicted use justify the price of the journal subscription? Does the journal deliver enough quality information on a page-by-page basis, per year, to justify a subscription? If the journal publishes only one or two high-quality or relevant articles per year, can the price be justified? A research study conducted by Schoch (1994) suggests that the higher cost of certain journals in a collection might not correlate with their perceived usefulness as measured by those particular journals that faculty actually have cited in their own publications (p. 37).

Usefulness of Journal Vendors

The majority of libraries do not buy their journal subscriptions directly from publishers. Although viewed with suspicion by some librarians, due to the perception that they may not always have the same interests in common with the libraries they serve, experience has proven the advantages of employing journals vendors (sometimes called serials vendors). The library normally contracts with the vendor to handle many of the activities for maintaining the subscription, such as placing orders, accounting for changed titles, and claiming undelivered issues from publishers. The library even may receive a discount from the vendor for contracting for a certain dollar amount of subscription purchases per year. The vendor gains from the relationship by using its large collective market share of placing many subscriptions from many libraries to individual publishers in exchange for a discount from the publisher. The vendor uses its large organization and knowledge of the journal publishing business to supply the aforementioned services to libraries more efficiently than the individual library could provide for itself.

The vendor's knowledge of the journal publishing business represents the greatest benefit to the collection development librarian. Vendors can provide customized reports that help the librarian manage the journals collection by tracking price increases historically by title, publisher, or subject area. The vendor can provide price inflation histories about journals under consideration as new subscriptions. Vendors also produce specialized subject lists of journals. The *Journals in Nursing* list produced by Bill Leazer (1996) at the vendor EBSCO serves as a noteworthy source for librarians selecting journals for nursing collections. In general, vendors can supply valuable information about predicted future price trends and observe patterns in the journals publishing marketplace through their many contacts in the industry that are not readily available to collection development librarians.

Electronic Journals

Ever since the prediction by F. W. Lancaster in 1978 that we were headed for "paperless information systems" (p. xi), librarians have envisioned the advent of electronic journals that, due to their faster delivery and superior capabilities of presenting information to readers, would replace print journals.

Conversely, Lewis (1995) and others have serious concerns about a library relinquishing access to all past issues in the event it cancels a subscription at a later date. Print journal subscriptions are "archived" in the collection even if the library cancels a journal subscription, whereas no guaranteed future access to archived electronic journals exists. In short, the promise of electronic journals remains unfulfilled, hampered by many unforeseen technical problems, especially relating to access, and economics, and so on. (Borghuis et al., 1996). Electronic nursing journals currently available are discussed in Chapter 1.

151

Jonathan DeForest Eldredge

Microforms

Libraries frequently occupy highly coveted physical space in their organizations; they also require a lot of space to store their collections. Thus, libraries or small collections located in clinical environments must compete with many other worthy functional work areas to remain easily accessible to their users. One technological solution that became popular in the 1950s and 1960s was the reproduction of printed texts on microfilm rolls, microfiche sheets, or microprint cards.

Although microforms provide high-density information in a small space, they have numerous disadvantages. Clinicians usually will refuse to use them due to the time constraints of setting up the equipment needed to read or copy the microforms. The equipment itself also takes some time to learn how to operate efficiently, although newer machines are more user-friendly. Furthermore, the equipment must be maintained; it requires space to house; and staff must be available to help clients with it. And the library still has to purchase a microfilm subscription to the journal, which represents yet another cost. Therefore, the cost savings versus added costs need to be weighed against the premium placed upon space at the institution. One option to consider is off-site storage of older volumes, although this, too, must be evaluated for the additional costs for storage, courier services, and personnel. Some libraries maintain older files of journals on microfilm. Weeding older and underutilized journal volumes, a subject discussed later in this chapter, may provide an even more practical solution.

Cancelations

The decision to cancel an existing subscription resembles the journal selection process of examining the merits of a journal itself, with one important difference. Because the institution already has made a significant investment in the journal by maintaining the subscription over the years, the clients' expectation to find the journal on the shelves in the future must be taken into account.

152

If the reason for the proposed journal cancelation stems from an apparent lack of use, this must be confirmed, because use of a particular journal title may fluctuate dramatically over several years. Judging a journal's use over too brief a period may simply record a lull rather than identify genuine low usage. The safest method to determine whether a journal has decreased in relevance is to contact those clients most likely to use the journal. Usually, they can offer a knowledgeable assessment for the decline in use. If the targeted clients point to a decline in the quality of the journal perhaps due to a change in editor, editorial board, governance, or publisher, probably the journal can be canceled. Schoch and Abels, (1994) provide an overview of other cancelation methods used in science libraries that might be applicable to health sciences collections, including citation analysis. Other major approaches and considerations in reviewing a journal's potential usefulness have been reviewed in the preceding pages.

BOOK SELECTION

Price Inflation

During the past decade, book prices have risen steadily, although the marketplace dynamics for books differs from those that have caused journal prices to rise over the same period due primarily to the different buying patterns practiced by most libraries. Where a journal subscription requires an advance payment from the library at least four months before the new subscription cycle begins, precluding the librarian having the opportunity to review the contents for the upcoming years' worth of the journal, many libraries receive much advance information about most books under consideration for purchase. Furthermore, many books may be obtained on a trial basis, then purchased on an approval plan, an option discussed later in this chapter. Should the librarian decide to not buy the book under consideration, it may be returned with no obligation. So while the same factors—peer review, editing, and production—cause price increases in book publishing, consumers can exercise greater flexibility in their purchasing decisions.

Jonathan DeForest Eldredge

Purposes of Books

Unfortunately, the greater inherent flexibility of the book selection process has prompted some libraries to reallocate their book budgets into their subscription budgets. This budgetary maneuver results in the purchase of few or no books, and signals a profound misunderstanding of the purposes served by books in most nursing collections.

In the broadest and not necessarily conventional use of the term, books primarily serve "educational" purposes. To the novice, a book is a concise introduction of a topic, concisely synthesizing much of the previous journal literature on the subject. Even in the age of electronic publishing, many students still rely on the textbook to become acquainted with a previously unknown subject. In the health sciences, particularly in this era of greater collaboration across disciplines, many experts in one field turn to books on a subject in which they hope to collaborate with others to grasp the essential principles of this new field. Experienced practitioners in a field also turn to recognized works, either to challenge their previous views, to update their professional knowledge bases in their own discipline, or for quick reference. Most books produced by reputable authors and publishers offer their readers bibliographic references that serve as expert guides to further reading on the subject.

Guides to Book Selection

Given the multidisciplinary sources of information accessed by nurses, a library's book selector needs to employ many different approaches to identifying and evaluating possible new titles for purchase. To aid in this task, this section reviews some of the more commonly utilized guides for selecting books, although the primary guide should always be the librarian's understanding of the interests and information needs of the customers.

Brandon-Hill Lists. When librarians refer to the Brandon-Hill List they almost always are specifying only one of three lists

154

by the same authors: the "Selected List of Books and Journals for the Small Medical Library" (Brandon & Hill, 1995). Although Brandon and Hill originally intended this list to be a book and journals selection guide for small hospital libraries, it now serves to some extent even large academic health sciences libraries. Slightly more than half (54 percent) of the respondents to a recent survey of academic health sciences libraries reported that they considered the Brandon-Hill List significantly influential (Murphy & Buchinger, 1996). This particular list has been mentioned by the Joint Commission on Accreditation of Healthcare Organizations standards in section 9.1 since 1994 (Joint Commission on Accreditation of Healthcare Organizations, 1996).

Items on the "Selected List of Nursing Books and Journals" (Brandon & Hill, 1994) may have greater utility on a title-by-title basis in developing a nursing collection. As its name implies, though, it focuses so narrowly upon nursing that it would be a disservice to use it exclusively for developing a nursing collection. A useful supplement to this list might be the Brandon Hill "Selected List of Books and Journals in Allied Health" (Brandon & Hill, 1996), which covers many subjects of shared interest and has a similar focus on patient contact shared between nurses and the allied health professions.

Lists of recommended books can bring to the attention of selectors titles that they may have previously overlooked. However, no list can be considered completely relevant to any library since the customers who use nursing collections can vary dramatically. And any selection process will be broadened and strengthened by drawing upon other professions' recommended lists rather than relying strictly upon "nursing only" titles.

Other Core Lists. The American College of Physicians has published a list of recommended books for practicing internists (Mazza, 1994), which is revised on a regular basis. Another core collection, although now dated, lists nursing books, journals, and media (Peretz, Stephan, & Terry, 1990).

Books of the Year. The January issue of *American Journal of Nursing* offers a select list of books chosen by recognized experts in their respective nursing specialties, including critical care, medical surgical, pediatric, and psychiatric nursing. Other categories cover education, research, and administration. The list for 1996 contains fewer than 40 titles, which limits its utility to the smallest collections. Regrettably, the sponsoring journal does not publicize the criteria employed by the expert judges for selecting the "best" books of the year, making it difficult to predict the value of individual titles at various locations.

Book Reviews. Most leading journals publish book reviews, which frequently reveal the criteria employed for making judgments about the quality of individual titles. These discussions also often describe the appropriate audiences for the book under review. The only disadvantage of book reviews, aside from the inevitable potential for reviewer bias, stems from the time lag between publication of the books and the appearance of their reviews. Reviews are most helpful for correcting deficiencies in specific subject areas in the collection. And book reviews in specialty journals are the obvious places to find evaluations of new books to supplement the more general book reviews found in mainstream journals.

The printed version of *Doody's Nursing and Allied Health Book Review Quarterly* reviews publications of interest to nurses. In addition, through a partnership effort between Doody Publishing, Login Brothers Book Company, and Sigma Theta Tau International (STTI) Honor Society for Nursing, the Sigma Theta Tau International Book Service is available to STTI members either in e-mail form or on the Web. It provides listings and peer reviews of newly published nursing books, and access to a database of books and software titles. Materials may be ordered electronically. A Personalized Weekly E-mail Bulletin automatically provides updates on new books and reviews in specialty areas.

Specialized Bibliographies. These specialized lists of books vary immensely, in number of references, criteria for inclusion, organization, and sponsorship; some contain annotations for listed books. Bibliographies may appear at the end of a book or journal article, or separately, as an equivalent of an article in a journal. Subject bibliographies on broad categories may be published as books unto themselves. The selector must ensure that any bibliographies employed for selection meet quality standards and have relevance for the customers who will use the specific nursing collection.

Vendors, too, produce subject bibliographies, which are generally helpful for initial identification of possible titles for selection. But before using such a resource it is essential to know the criteria for inclusion of the specific titles. Many vendors now offer online databases of their book titles, which allow for creating individual subject bibliographies of in-print books. The selector usually can be assured of the availability from the vendor of any titles generated by these database searches. The National Library of Medicine's CATLINE database allows the selector to create subject bibliographies containing many of the known English-language books on the subject for recent years.

Essential Nursing References (Interagency Council on Information Resources for Nursing, 1996), published biennially, lists many types of reference sources covering a broad range of topics, including general biomedical sources as well as those specific to nursing.

Regular features in the printed *International Nursing Index* include "Nursing-Related Data Sources," a listing of recent studies and surveys directly related to nursing; "Publications of Organizations and Agencies"; and "Nursing Books Published," although none of the titles listed in these bibliographies are evaluated.

Existing Collections. The holdings of another library, particularly if there are similarities in client bases between the two institutions, can prove to be a valuable aid to book selection. By examining recent additions to the larger library's collection, a librarian may find titles suitable for his or her own library. In the absence of complete holdings on the shelf, the librarian utilizing this approach needs to obtain a complete list of recently published titles to avoid having a distorted view of holdings and possibly missing the most relevant and potentially popular titles.

A variation of this approach is to search another library's Online Public Access Catalog via the Internet. But while more convenient, the selector cannot actually examine and read portions of the titles, limiting the quality of the information—although increasingly tables of contents are attached to cataloging records in online catalogs, partially reducing this deficiency. But when the selector knows little about the publisher, author, or the subject, reviewing tables of contents online also has its limitations.

Publishers' Flyers and Catalogs. Promotional materials can be immensely valuable not only to identify potential purchases but to find descriptions of contents of the books as well. The larger health sciences book vendors and publishers produce substantial book catalogs arranged in subject categories, which enable the collection development librarian to quickly compare titles available with those already owned in specific subject areas.

That said, catalogs and flyers sometimes omit crucial information about a book. For example, a conference proceeding may not be indicated as such in promotional material. And promotional materials also tend to saturate the recipient with information about familiar books. Major health sciences publishers are prolific in such mailings. Nevertheless, the discriminating recipient often can cull these mailings from the small, underrepresented health sciences publishers, the foreign publishers, or those publishers that normally do not publish much in the health sciences. This is important because these mailings may be the only reliable method of learning about high-quality books not published by the large mainstream health sciences companies.

Approval Plans. A library that can allocate thousands or tens of thousands of dollars to books each year may want to utilize an approval plan offered by the major health sciences book vendors. Such a plan enables the library to design a profile of the subject matter, publishers, and formats (textbooks, handbooks, exam review guides) that it would like to receive automatically from the vendor. Some profiles are very broad, and the library will receive an entire subject class of books, while other profiles let the library specify exactly the types of books it wants to receive automatically. Practices vary, but under most approval plans, the library receives the books in the predetermined profile each week, and is given a two-week review period. Rejected books are returned to the vendor without cost.

Certainly an approval plan concept has great appeal due to convenience and simplicity, but the collection development librarian must be vigilant to ensure that all books fitting the profile are sent to the library. Most vendors share information on all books received during the week so these lists can be compared for possible omissions. In addition, a library utilizing such a plan will sometimes be allowed to select books not fitting the profile, when circumstances dictate. Also, some vendors list online both their weekly shipment of approval books and those books not fitting the profile. By reviewing these online lists, books may be selected or eliminated prior to shipment, saving the vendor and the library valuable time and energy.

One word of caution: Vendors may sever their relationships with publishers without notice, so selecting a publisher using a predetermined profile does not guarantee that books produced by that publisher will be automatically sent to the library in the future. Again, vigilance will detect discrepancies and gaps.

Associations That Publish

Associations that publish represent one of the most valuable sources of books. Eldredge (1996) provides a list of nearly 300 associations that publish on subjects with relevance to the health sciences, and 21 specialty and other nursing associations that publish books or other significant publications identified in this article are included in Appendix C.

Unfortunately, associations often publish only for their members, and only as a membership benefit, so normal customer service conventions practiced by commercial publishers may be largely absent. These absent amenities may lead to customer frustration and confusion.

Fortunately, the National League for Nursing (NLN) and the American Nurses Association (ANA) have major publishing programs, and both offer standing order programs to enable a library to receive all of their publications automatically. NLN and ANA also publish practice standards and guidelines, and tend to publish reports and books on highly relevant contemporary issues in nursing or on public policy issues affecting the nursing profession. NLN emphasizes education directories for undergraduate and graduate study programs, curriculum guides, career guides, statistical data compilations, and subjects such as nursing research and Total Quality Management (TQM). ANA publishes on credentialing matters, quality indicators, and guidelines. ANA also occasionally publishes symposia proceedings.

Special Types of Monographs

Government Publications. Many government agencies at the federal, state, county, and local levels produce documents of interest to the clientele of health sciences libraries. Even quasi-governmental entities such as the United Nations and the World Health Organization produce documents concerning the health sciences.

Many librarians associate the phrase "government document" with the Government Printing Office (GPO), a federal system for distributing and storing documents around the country to ensure access to U.S. government agency publications. Libraries that make these documents available to the public are known as depositories in the GPO system. The GPO has been undergoing major changes in recent years, with many more anticipated in the near future, principally revolving around the issues of electronic access to these documents. Within a decade, the local GPO depository collection consisting of printed materials may be replaced by electronic Web sites (Flagg, 1996).

Federal agencies sometimes produce documents that are not part of the GPO depository program. These pose a challenge to identify and locate. The health departments at state, county, and local levels of government, too, can provide valuable information nowhere else available. These documents also tend to be difficult to identify and obtain from publishing agencies. Having a contact inside these agencies, or a sympathetic elected representative often facilitates this process. Be prepared to pay a fee to the issuing agency as a cost-recovery measure. (Additional information on government publications is included in Chapter 4.)

Textbooks. There are three basic types of textbooks published: the programmed text, the introductory text, and the authoritative core textbook. Most libraries avoid the programmed textbooks since they serve as interactive guides for students as they proceed through a course, and inevitably become defaced by students' writings or have pages removed. Review guides intended to prepare students for national boards such as NCLEX are not kept by many libraries for the same reason. Introductory textbooks, sometimes known as "can openers," often provide such elementary treatment of a subject that they too are not useful for libraries.

The third type, the core textbook, is the only type of textbook actively collected by most libraries. A core textbook will be most useful to an advanced student in the subject area, a practitioner in the profession, or a faculty member. It serves as an authoritative source for updating the knowledge base of someone already well-acquainted with the field or for quickly looking up specific information. Many times, the latest edition of one or two core textbooks per field should suffice for clients' needs in a library.

Handbooks. Practitioners or advanced trainees in a professional health care degree program find pocket-sized or slightly larger handbooks helpful to carry in their lab coats or with their files when they see patients. Larger libraries normally do not collect these since they are best utilized near the patient care arena, but these handbooks are popular when added to small collections at nursing stations or in call rooms. As a general rule, handbooks are most appropriate for patient care settings.

Practice Guidelines. While most health care professionals will agree that certain patient care guidelines are important for providing standard care for patients, in recent years controversy has emerged concerning their use. Some health care providers worry that too-strict adherence to practice guidelines leads to "robot health care," which is the antithesis of professionalism. Others are concerned that too much latitude by professionals may undermine accountability in practice. The collection development librarian needs to be aware of the general consensus about the use of practice guidelines among library clientele, and they should be selected for relevant subject areas only to the extent that they are valued by clientele. Practice guidelines may appear as separate documents, features in journals, or as part of compilations. A great many professional associations also publish practice guidelines. Some are also available in HSTAT (Health Services/Technology Assessment Text); access: http://text.nlm.nih.gov/.

Consumer Health and Patient Guides. Many contemporary patients expect to be educated about their medical condition; their relatives or other caregivers often want to learn all that may be practical about the patient's condition as well. To meet this growing demand, a clinical area may provide patients with a small collection of books written for the layperson regarding common diseases or conditions treated in that clinic. Patient guides, generally available in pamphlet form, may be distributed by physicians or nurses to interested patients.

Some hospitals are establishing patient education centers where patients and their caregivers may learn more about the pertinent disease or condition. Even libraries serving large health sciences centers make consumer health books available to the public. Broering (1996) indicates: "Health sciences librarians are the most knowledgeable and prominent professionals prepared to provide information to the public" (p. 237). The Medical Library Association (1996) has outlined the roles of the librarians in the provision of consumer health information. The major book selection challenges concerning these consumer health collections are twofold: determining which diseases or conditions need to be covered; and identifying which books are most authoritative and yet easy to comprehend by the person with no health care training. The predominant 50 to 100 Diagnostic Related Groups (DRGs) of the nearby health care facilities, knowledge of the incidence and prevalence of major health conditions in the general population, and questions previously asked at the library will provide help in addressing the first of the two major challenges of book selection.

Experience in assisting those people seeking consumer health information will be one of the greatest aids in determining subjects of greatest relevance to include in the collection.

The second challenge, identifying authoritative books to house in your collection, will require some effort. The best sources are book reviews in the leading professional journals although they tend to cover books already in print for a year or two. Some health sciences book vendors publish and make available subject guides to consumer health books (Majors Scientific Books, 1996c; Rittenhouse Book Distributors, 1996). These subject guides are fairly comprehensive, but do not provide the quality-filtering dimension available from book reviews. (Additional information on patient and consumer information is included in Chapter 4.)

GIFTS ADMINISTRATION

Rapid changes in the health sciences generally leads to high rates of obsolescence for published information, thus the vast majority of books and journals over 10 years old that are offered as gifts for addition to a collection consequently will be useless. Still, a library with any sort of goal concerning the collection of materials for historical purposes will have to accept gifts, in order to acquire otherwise unavailable or expensive titles. With these constraints in mind, a gifts policy should clearly state that receivership of donated items in no way obligates the library to add these items to the collection, or to retain indefinitely any items added to the collection. Parent institutions may also have policies governing the receipt of gifts that will have to be applied consistently to gifts to the library.

Although the evaluation of gifts normally is of a low priority in most health sciences libraries, at the very least, gifts should be acknowledged through a telephone call, e-mail, or letter within a few days. A letter probably should tactfully state the gifts policy so that the donor is not misled or mistaken about the fate of donated items. Often, books donated are in turn donated to an annual book sale for raising funds for the library. Donors should be informed of the likelihood that their donation will be handled in this way. Offers for donations of journals normally are referred to

163

hospital or departmental libraries that may be able to use these titles to enhance their collections. Occasionally, bound journals that have been donated may be used to replace worn volumes, at least in the cases of heavily used titles. Otherwise, unsolicited journals that are donated may be used in an exchange program or recycled.

Needless to say, donor subscriptions to journals needed by the library are an important exception to the preceding generalizations. The gifts policy should state that the donor will be invoiced by the publisher or vendor, but that the journal(s) will be directly mailed from the publisher or vendor to the library.

If the aforementioned guidelines seem unnecessarily harsh and perhaps rigid to nonlibrarians or inexperienced librarians, it is important to recognize that there are no free "gifts"; often, the time required to handle, evaluate, and process any donated materials can exceed the purchase price of new materials. These value-added processes by libraries, whether for new or donated materials, enable customers to obtain useful information from collections.

ELECTRONIC RESOURCES AND NEW MEDIA SELECTION

While electronic journals may not replace print journals in the foreseeable future (Clark, 1997), some exciting new innovations are occurring in other applications of information technology. Internet searches for information constitute one of the most high-profile and popular applications. Searches that yield Web sites of interest can be bookmarked by libraries for future reference for clients to supplement information available through on-site collections. Web sites have limitations, however. Many times, they provide little information beyond that found in a directory or a print brochure, and the quality of the information can vary dramatically between sites. Rioux (1996) cautions that much of the information found at Web sites becomes dated quickly. She also warns users to be highly skeptical of the reliability of information obtained on the Internet. In contrast, print sources have developed mechanisms over the years for ensuring quality of the information presented.

Alling (1996) has clustered the new electronic media used on-site into three basic groupings: testing software; reference software; and multimedia. Alling views these new media as potentially superior for meeting the need for ready access to information. These new media are most likely to be popular with students who find it more effective to learn when sound and video are incorporated into the presentation of text.

The first type of new media, testing software, provides instant feedback to users about their performance. Testing software also compiles a profile on the user's strengths and weaknesses so the student can prioritize study time for maximum results. Most libraries do not provide student review guides for national exams because these print materials are prone to damage by students who deface or remove pages, and the new testing software may eliminate or reduce these problems. But a common, and still unalleviated drawback of both print review guides and the new media testing software is the heavy demand for the same resources by numerous students.

Reference software enables the user to enjoy all of the benefits of print textbooks with the added capability of automatic searching by keywords. Furthermore, reference software may combine the contents of textbooks with other reference guides that students may want to access. Alling writes: "For example, you can search across a medical-surgical nursing reference and a drug handbook at the same time for a particular drug name" (p. 5). Alling cautions, however, that "products still vary in quality" (p. 5) so the selector needs to carefully review the software before purchasing.

The third type of new media, termed multimedia by Alling, combines many of the advantages of the previous two categories while incorporating "sound, video, animation, and still pictures in addition to standard text" (p. 6). Again, he warns readers to be careful when selecting these new media due to varying quality.

The Bosch, Promis, and Sugnet's (1994) guide published by the American Library Association, introduces the selector to the many types of nonprint media available on the market, and offers criteria for selection, along with information on common pitfalls, licensing agreements, and copyright issues. The new media will most likely be of greatest use to collections serving an educational mission.

WEEDING COLLECTIONS

Ironically, the appropriate weeding of collections normally increases the use of remaining materials (Slote, 1989). Weeding consists of the systematic effort to remove materials from the shelves that reasonably can be judged as no longer useful to customers. But weeded materials are not necessarily tossed into a dumpster; they may be offered to other libraries or moved to an off-site storage space so that they may still be accessed, but do not clutter up crowded shelves in the publicly accessible collection. This ease of access leads to greater use of the collection.

Weeding a collection should be systematic, rational, and provide an opportunity for dialogue with potentially affected individuals (Saar, 1996). It should not be undertaken unilaterally or without agreed-upon criteria (Baker, 1996).

A retention policy can reduce the recurring need to weed a collection. Ask: Does your collection need to own all past editions of textbooks? For example, the author's library retains "classic core collection" titles consisting of the most respected textbook at the time of publication so that researchers might refer to these for historical comparison. Earlier editions of nursing textbooks make for fascinating reading and point to the advances of the field, but access to historical texts may not be a priority. And space limitations force hard choices in setting priorities.

Similarly, you need to determine whether all journals should be kept indefinitely. Use studies of your collection or the citation analysis of references used by library clientele may indicate an effective shelf life of journals lasting only 5 to 10 years. Access to older volumes of certain journals can be guaranteed through interlibrary loan, so there may be no need to retain these titles in the collection. Notable exceptions may include *Nursing* or *American Journal of Nursing,* and possibly the *New England Journal of Medicine* or *JAMA: Journal of the American Medical Association.*

166

Certain journals and their articles are often rediscovered or still found useful many years after their initial publication.

COLLECTION ASSESSMENT AND EVALUATION

Assessment and evaluation projects tend to be complicated and time-consuming when executed on a broad scale encompassing entire collections. Yet most libraries conduct far more modest microassessments and microevaluations every day. Clients assess and evaluate collections every time they utilize their libraries. Whenever clients search for specific books or research defined subjects, they evaluate the quality of collections. Thus, staying in close contact with clientele increases the likelihood that librarians will hear these evaluations and factor them into their selection activities.

An accreditation process for programs by external reviewers and formation of new programs will provide the most common occasions for collection assessment and evaluation. An accreditation process every several years by the Joint Commission for the Accreditation of Healthcare Organizations (JCAHO), or other organizations that evaluate clinical programs, provides another opportunity to assess and evaluate collections. The beginning of or expansion of new programs in need of library service present another opportunity for assessing and evaluating collections in subjects relevant to the new program.

Collection Assessment

Assessment and evaluation are often mentioned in the same breath, and incorrectly used interchangeably due to their close connection in a review process of collections. *Assessment* technically involves a description of a collection. An assessment may produce a descriptive profile of subjects that are emphasized in the overall collection when conducted on a broad scale. More commonly, the assessment describes the areas of emphasis or relative lack of emphasis in a more narrowly defined subject area of the collection. Collection assessment should not be confused with collection audits that determine to what extent a collection contains the titles it acquired has been dimished due to theft (Kiger & Wise, 1996).

Assessment does not make judgments about the efficacy of the collection per se, but rather establishes the map for the evaluation to follow. The goals of the collection evaluation project frequently determine how the collection profile will be defined in an assessment profile. For example, in a field in which currency of the literature will be vitally important, the age of the collection will be an integral part of the collection assessment profile. Collection evaluation utilizes the description produced from the assessment phase to compare the collection with carefully defined standards.

Assessment may take many forms. A global assessment looks at the areas of relative emphases in the overall collection, and normally profiles these emphases by quantifying the holdings in each National Library of Medicine classification category (QT, QZ, W, WC, WO, WY, etc.) or, if applicable, the Library of Congress classification schedule categories (Rs for the health sciences). These categories may be analyzed in terms of the age of holdings in these broad subject areas. For example, molecular biology or cell biology holdings may be analyzed by age since their literatures are rapidly changing to reflect their fields; thus, currency may be important. A specific collection evaluation goal would be implied by such a narrowly defined assessment. Currency of the collection may not be as important in subject areas such as anatomy, history, or theory. A downside to global assessments is that they may invite dangerous comparisons between broad subject classes, since these classification schemes are limited in their ability to define subject areas in ways that researchers and clinicians actually conceptualize their fields. The fact that medical-surgical nursing monographs outnumber community nursing or pediatric nursing monographs in the collection by a 4 to 1 and 2 to 1 ratio, respectively, may not form a significant basis for conducting an evaluation either. Linking expenditures in recent years to broad subject classifications can be hazardous, too, since unit prices per title vary according to subject area, and some subject areas are overrepresented by publisher productivity in certain years (Majors Scientific Books, 1996a).

Collection assessments may compare specific titles in the collection with titles on a select or authoritative bibliography. In nursing, comparing collection holdings to either the Brandon-Hill "Selected List of Nursing Books and Journals" (Brandon & Hill, 1994) or the annual "Books of the Year" list in the *American Journal of Nursing* is probably the most popular assessment activity. In the absence of specific collection evaluation goals, based on an understanding of the mission of the institution and customer needs, such superficial assessments increase the risk of making inappropriate comparisons. For example, would a graduate nursing program want to have its collections judged by whether or not it contained textbooks on the Brandon-Hill list intended for practicing LPNs or RNs? Most likely, it would not.

Emerging subject areas for which no select or authoritative lists exist may be aided by the Landmark Citation Method developed by Soehner, Wray, and Richards (1992). This method relies upon selecting a key article and tracking the articles and books that cite this article in subsequent years. It was developed for the new field of biotechnology, and relied upon tools such as *Science Citation Index*. The value of this approach could be of benefit in new subject areas of interest to nurses.

The conspectus approach to assessment compares collection holdings of unique titles to those at peer institutions, forming the basis for a "collection centered evaluation" described next. Although developed and normally used for comparing large research libraries, White (1995) indicates that the methods could be applied in other types of libraries. The possibilities are compelling. One could identify leading institutions that share an emphasis upon a common subject area such as gerontological nursing and then compare one's collection strength (measured by number of titles and perhaps their relative recency) to the same assessments of other collections. These types of conspectus studies assume that different institutions share enough common characteristics to be meaningfully considered peers. The presence of a unique title at a peer library moreover does not signal that it exhibits sufficient quality to have been acquired in the first place! In an era in which no one collection can hope to purchase all desired titles, some librarians suggest that the conspectus approach can assist in cooperative collection development projects that increase the likelihood that at least one participating library in a consortium might own all desired titles (Allen, 1995).

Collection Evaluation

Richards (1991) has categorized collection evaluation activities into two distinctly different approaches: collection-centered and use-centered (pp. 54–55).

Collection-centered approaches, as the term implies, focus upon the collection and possibly how the collection might be compared to other collections or standards of quality for collections. The bibliographic comparison method, described in the previous discussion of assessments, attempts to evaluate collection holdings when compared to authoritative inventories such as the Brandon-Hill (1994) list or the "Books of the Year" lists published in the *American Journal of Nursing*. These authoritative lists need to be relevant to the goals of the institution and the needs of clients, however. The conspectus approach, just described, represents another type of collection-centered evaluation technique when meaningful inferences can be made by comparing peer libraries.

Collections may be evaluated by experts, who normally are recognized authorities in at least the bibliography of the field, if not experts in the field itself. These projects are expensive and time-consuming unless perhaps the subject area under evaluation consists of fewer than 200 titles. Library clientele might serve as experts provided they can provide an objective evaluation that does not just reflect their own particular and narrow interests in viewing what should be in the collection.

Global assessments may provide the raw data for evaluating collection strength. Nursing has a strong multidisciplinary orientation to the health sciences literature. Nevertheless, if a global assessment produces a profile suggesting that nursing (WY in the

National Library of Medicine classification) represents only 10 percent of a collection intended solely for supporting a nursing program, an evaluation can safely state that nursing has been underrepresented in the collection—at least, provided there are no local circumstances that might explain such an unusual profile. Assessments of subject emphases within a nursing collection may produce a profile of books published within the past five years in which psychiatric nursing has 10 times as many titles as medical-surgical nursing titles that have been published in the past five years. But the medical-surgical nurses in the clinical areas or the medical-surgical nursing students might outnumber psychiatric nursing students or practitioners by a ratio of 10 to 1. Carrigan (1996a) indicates that many times evaluation methods focus upon deficiencies but do not recognize the existence of overselection in certain subjects, which consequently have robbed the underrepresented subjects of adequate holdings (pp. 273–274). In this instance, medical-surgical nursing might have been benefited by better representation by more recent literature due to rapid changes in that field. Rao (1993) has reminded her readers of the frequent need to examine the currency of holdings in a collection as one possible element in collection evaluation. In all of these collection-centered approaches, there may be local circumstances created by customers that might explain irregularities in any comparisons between the collection and other sources or collections. Collection-centered approaches offer the advantage of producing a starting point by identifying possible problem areas that may or may not be explained by the use-centered methods of evaluation, described next.

Use-Centered Approaches. Client preferences, as expressed through use-centered approaches to collection evaluation, provide a compelling argument for either validating current selection activities or for making changes in the types of items selected. Circulation studies are the most popular form of use-centered approaches to collection evaluation. The advent of sophisticated software for creating reports from online circulation systems has greatly facilitated what used to require great investments of personnel resources to conduct circulation studies manually. Atkins

(1996) asserts: "It is almost a crime how little this capacity has been utilized," although Carrigan (1996b) has determined that there are many practical constraints to utilizing these reports more fully (pp. 434–436). Ideally, both in-house use of materials and actual checkouts will be measured in a circulation study. Walters (1996) recently reported that in-house use at a major health sciences center library overshadowed checkouts by ratios ranging 4 to 16 depending upon the subject area. Many library clients never check out materials so this in-house usage needs to be measured.

Circulation studies sometimes reveal that only a small percentage of the collection may account for a large percentage of what clients actually use (Kent, 1979). The so-called 80/20 rule expressed this concept when it was discovered that 80 percent of the usage at certain large academic research libraries could be linked to only 20 percent of the collection. Britten (1990) uncovered major deviations from this rule when he determined that the ratio of use to nonuse fluctuated widely according to subject areas. Using both in-house and external checkouts, it may be determined that a large percentage of the monographs circulate each year, and that most titles acquired within the past five years experienced use. A more detailed examination of collection use for discrete subject areas may uncover "thin" areas in which the collection appeared to have too few monographs to handle the high circulation figures linked to those subjects. Shelf availability studies in which certain subjects are consistently used, and thereby missing from the shelves, achieve the same objectives for determining subject deficiencies within the collection in the absence of sophisticated circulation report software. Regardless of approach, circulation studies almost always reveal surprising information on how library clientele use the collection.

Interlibrary loan studies sometimes produce surprising results about which subjects may be underrepresented in the collection. The journals selection section discussed using interlibrary loan records to determine which journal titles are consistently requested from other libraries. Interlibrary loan records also may produce trends in subjects repeatedly sought from other libraries, apparently when local collection resources were inadequate. This approach may sometimes produce very few subject areas that might need strengthening in the collection. In fact, such a study could show a high correlation between heavy interlibrary loan use and heavy representation in the existing collection for a majority of subjects!

Citation analysis in collection evaluation will be most applicable to academic health sciences libraries where a great many library clients publish their research. By linking the works cited by these faculty authors in their publications, one can evaluate how helpful the on-site collection turned out to be in fulfilling faculty needs for works considered important enough to cite in their publications. This approach to collection evaluation may uncover important journal titles or monographs that perhaps should be owned by the library. A variation of this approach simply links the titles in which clients publish to what exists in the collection. If a faculty member publishes more than once in an unowned journal, it might raise the possibility that the journal would be a useful addition to the collection. This more detailed form of citation analysis can be very tedious and the results not always easy to interpret for selection goals.

Use-centered collection evaluation tends to be favored by many librarians because these approaches attempt to understand what clients really need. Use-centered approaches have some limitations that should be kept in mind, however. What clients have used in the collection cannot be linked necessarily to a definition of quality. Convergently, what clients have used cannot be equated with client satisfaction either. In addition, past use of the collection should never be translated into inevitable predictions about what will be used in the future since programs and the interests of clients continuously change.

CONCLUSION

Collection development and evaluation follow an iterative process of assessing primary clientele needs, selecting quality information resources to meet those needs, and evaluating the success by which these efforts meet their objectives. Continuous and close contact with nurses, nursing students, faculty, or practitioners to facilitate healthy communication represents a time-tested, low-cost method of assessing needs.

REFERENCES

Allen, B. M. (1995). Theoretical value of conspectus-based (cooperative) collection management. *Collection Building, 13,* 7–10.

Alling, J. (1996). A 10-minute guide to new media and the health sciences. *Rittenhouse Quarterly Report, 1*(3), 3–9.

Atkins, S. (1996). Mining automated systems for collection management. *Library Administration & Management, 10,* 16–19.

Baker, N. (1996, October 14). The author vs. the library. *New Yorker, 72,* 50–62.

Blythe, J., & Royle, J. A. (1993). Assessing nurses' information needs in the work environment. *Bulletin of the Medical Library Association, 81,* 433–435.

Books of the year. (1996). *American Journal of Nursing, 96,* 50–51.

Borghuis, M., Brinckman, H., Fischer, A., Hunter, K., van der Loo, E., Mors, R. T., Mostert, P., & Zijlstra, J. (Contr.). (1996, July 18). *TULIP: Final report.* (The University Licensing Program) (www.elsevier.nl.80 /homepage/about/resproj/trmenu.htm). New York: Elsevier.

Bosch, S., Promis, P., & Sugnet, C. (1994). *Guide to selecting and acquiring CD-ROMs, software and other electronic publications.* Chicago: American Library Association.

Brandon A. N., & Hill, D. R. (1979). Selected list of nursing books and journals. *Nursing Outlook, 27,* 672–680.

Brandon, A. N., & Hill, D. R. (1994). Selected list of nursing books and journals. *Nursing Outlook, 42,* 71–82.

Brandon, A. N., & Hill, D. R. (1995). Selected list of books and journals for the small medical library. *Bulletin of the Medical Library Association, 83,* 151–175.

Brandon, A. N., & Hill, D. R. (1996). Selected list of books and journals in allied health. *Bulletin of the Medical Library Association, 84,* 289–309.

Britten, W. A. (1990). A use of statistics for collection management: The 80/20 rule revisited. *Library Acquisitions: Practice & Theory, 14,* 183–189.

Broering, N. C. (1996). Highlighting consumer health information. *Bulletin of the Medical Library Association, 84,* 237.

Bruwelheide, J. H. (1995). *The copyright primer for librarians and educators* (2nd ed.). Chicago: American Library Association; Washington, DC: National Education Association.

174

Burdick, A. J., Butler, A., & Sullivan, M. G. (1993). Citation patterns in the health sciences: Implications for serials/monographic fund allocation. *Bulletin of the Medical Library Association, 81,* 44–47.

Burnham, J. C. (1990). The evolution of editorial peer review. *JAMA: Journal of the American Medical Association, 263,* 1323–1329.

Cargill, J. (1984). Collection development policies: An alternative viewpoint. *Library Acquisitions: Practice and Theory, 8,* 47–49.

Carpenter, E. J. (1984). Collection development policies: The case for. *Library Acquisitions: Practice and Theory, 8,* 43–45.

Carrigan, D. P. (1996a). Collection development—evaluation. *Journal of Academic Librarianship, 22,* 273–278.

Carrigan, D. P. (1996b). Data-guided collection development: A promise unfulfilled. *College & Research Libraries, 57,* 429–438.

Clark, D. (1997, January 14). Facing early losses, some Web publishers begin to pull the plug. *Wall Street Journal, 136*(9), 1, 9.

Cohn, S., Brondoli, M., & Bedell, M. (1996). If publishers perished, just what would be lost? *Serials Librarian, 28,* 371–375.

Colglazier, M. L. (1996). The causal relationship between clinical activity and journal use in a hospital library as analyzed by multiple regression. *Bulletin of the Medical Library Association, 84,* 569–571.

Delman, B. S. (1982). A problem-oriented approach to journal selection for hospital libraries. *Bulletin of the Medical Library Association, 70,* 397–410.

Eakin, D. (1993). A review column is born. *Serials Review, 19,* 41–44.

Eldredge, J. D. (1996). Associations that produce significant publications for the health sciences: Results from tracking a phantom literature. *Bulletin of the Medical Library Association, 84,* 572–578.

Eldredge, J. D. (1997, February). JAMA journal reviews: Analysis and master index: 1992–1996. *MLA News* (293), 22–24.

Flagg, G. (1996, October). GPO proposes changes to federal depository program. *American Libraries,* 11.

Garfield, E. (1996, September 2). The significant scientific literature appears in a small core of journals. *The Scientist, 10*(17), 1, 16.

Garfield, E. (1972). Citation analysis as a tool in journal evaluation. *Science, 178,* 471–479.

Henderson, A. (1995). Solving the paradoxes of journals prices: An editor's response to the serials crisis. *CBE Views, 18,* 31–35.

Interagency Council on Information Resources for Nursing. (1996). Essential nursing references. *N&HC Perspectives on Community, 17,* 255–259.

Joint Commission on Accreditation of Healthcare Organizations. (1996). *Comprehensive accreditation manual for hospitals: The official handbook.* Oakbrook Terrace, IL: Joint Commission.

Kent, A. (1979). *Use of library materials: The University of Pittsburgh study.* New York: Dekker.

Kiger, J. E., & Wise, K. (1996). Auditing an academic library book collection. *Journal of Academic Librarianship, 22,* 267–272.

Lacroix, E. M. (1994). Interlibrary loan in U.S. health sciences libraries: Journal article use. *Bulletin of the Medical Library Association, 82,* 363–368.

Lancaster, F. W. (1978). *Toward paperless information systems.* New York: Academic Press.

Leazer, B. (Comp.). (1996). *Journals in nursing, 1996.* Birmingham, AL: Ebsco.

Lewis, D. W. (1989). Economics of the scholarly journal. *College & Research Libraries, 50,* 674–688.

Lewis, S. (1995). From earth to ether: One publisher's reincarnation. *Serials Librarian, 25,* 173–180.

Majors Scientific Books. (1996a). *Ten-year statistical analysis by categories 1985–1994.* Dallas: Majors Scientific Books.

Majors Scientific Books. (1996b). *Ten-year statistical analysis by publishers 1985–1994.* Dallas: Majors Scientific Books.

Majors Scientific Books. (1996c). *Consumer Health Books.* Dallas: Majors Scientific Books.

Marshall, J. G. (1992). The impact of the hospital library on clinical decision making: The Rochester study. *Bulletin of the Medical Library Association, 80,* 169–178.

Mazza, J. J. (1994). A library for internists VIII. *Annals of Internal Medicine, 120,* 699–720.

McClure, L. W. (1995). MLA and AAHSLD testimony on intellectual property and the national information infrastructure. *Bulletin of the Medical Library Association, 83,* 252–253.

Medical Library Association. (1996). The librarian's role in the provision of consumer health information and patient education. *Bulletin of the Medical Library Association, 84,* 238–239.

Murphy, S. C., & Buchinger, K. (1996). Academic health sciences librarians' use of the Brandon-Hill selected list in book selection activities: Results of a preliminary descriptive study. *Bulletin of the Medical Library Association, 84,* 427–431.

Peretz, A., Stephan, A., & Terry, E. (1990). *Core collection in nursing and the allied health sciences:* Books, journals, media. Phoenix, AZ: Oryx Press.

Rao, S. N. (1993). Meeting modern demands of collection evaluation: A new approach. *Collection Building, 13,* 33–36.

Richards, D. T. (1991). *Development and assessment of health sciences library collections.* CE 701. Course for Continuing Education Syllabus. Chicago: Medical Library Association.

Rioux, M. A. (1996, June). *Order out of chaos: Collection development and management of Internet resources: Hunting and gathering in cyberspace* (Concurrent Session). North American Serials Interest Group (NASIG), 11th Annual Conference, Albuquerque, NM.

Rittenhouse Book Distributors. (1996). *Consumer health books, 1996–1997.* King of Prussia, PA: Rittenhouse Book.

Roche, M. M. (1993). *ARL/RLG interlibrary loan cost study.* Washington, DC: Association of Research Libraries.

Rousseau, R., & Van Hooydonk, G. (1996). Journal production and journal impact factors. *Journal of the American Society for Information Science, 47,* 775–780.

Saar, A. E. F. (1996, October). *Storage, weeding, and the process of grieving: Not making change any easier than it has to be.* Paper presentation at the Medical Library Association South Central Chapter Annual Meeting. Galveston, TX.

Schoch, N. (1994). Relationship between citation frequency and journal cost: A comparison between pure and applied science disciplines. *Proceedings of the 57th annual meeting of the American Society for Information Science, 31,* 34–40.

Schoch, N., & Abels, E. G. (1994). Using a valuative instrument for decision making in the cancellation of science journals in a university setting. *Proceedings of the 57th annual meeting of the American Society for Information Science, 31,* 41–47.

Sievert, M. E., McKinin, E. J., Johnson, E. D., Reid, J. C., & Mitchell, J. A. (1996). Beyond relevance—characteristics of key papers for clinicians: An exploratory study in an academic setting. *Bulletin of the Medical Library Association, 84,* 351–357.

Slote, S. J. (1989). *Weeding library collections* (3rd ed.). Englewood, CO: Libraries Unlimited Inc.

Snow, B. (1996) Wasted words: The written collection development policy and the academic library. *Journal of Academic Librarianship, 22,* 191–194.

Soehner, C. B., Wray, S. T., & Richards, D. T. (1992). The landmark citation method: Analysis of a citation pattern as a collection assessment method. *Bulletin of the Medical Library Association, 80,* 361–366.

Walters, P. L. (1996). A journal use study: Checkouts and in house use. *Bulletin of the Medical Library Association, 84,* 461–467.

White, H. D. (1995). *Brief tests of collection strength: A methodology for all types of libraries.* Westport, CT: Greenwood Press.

Weaver, S. M. (1993). Information literacy: Educating for life-long learning. *Nurse Educator, 18,* 30–32.

RESOURCE REFERENCES

Bosch, S., Promis, P., & Sugnet, C. (1994). *Guide to selecting and acquiring CD-ROMs, software, and other electronic publications.* Chicago: American Library Association.

177

Eldredge, J. D. (1996). Associations that produce significant publications for the health sciences: Results from tracking a phantom literature. *Bulletin of the Medical Library Association, 84,* 572–578.

Evans, G. E. (1987). *Developing library and information center collections* (2nd ed.). Littleton, CO: Libraries Unlimited.

Futas, E. (1995). *Collection development policies and procedures.* Phoenix, AZ: Oryx Press.

Interagency Council on Information Resources for Nursing. (1996). Essential nursing references. *N&HC Perspectives on Community, 17,* 255–259.

Martin, M. S. (1995). *Collection development and finance: A guide to strategic library-materials budgeting.* Chicago: American Library Association.

Robinson, J. S. (1993). *Tapping the government grapevine: the user-friendly guide to U. S. government information sources* (2nd ed.). Phoenix, AZ: Oryx Press.

Sarazen, J. S., & Salter, J. M. (1993). *Managing the customer satisfaction process.* Watertown, MA: American Management Association.

Slote, S. J. (1989). *Weeding library collections* (3rd ed.). Englewood, CO: Libraries Unlimited.

SUGGESTED READINGS

Alling, J. (1996). A 10-minute guide to new media and the health sciences. *Rittenhouse Quarterly Report, 1*(3), 3–9.

Carpenter, K. H., & Alexander, A. W. (1996, May). U.S. periodical price index for 1996. *American Libraries, 27,* 97–105.

Carrigan, D. P. (1995). Toward a theory of collection development. *Library Acquisitions: Practice and Theory, 19,* 97–106.

Chrzastowski, T. E., & Stern, D. (1994). Duplicate serial subscriptions: Can use justify the cost of duplication? *Serials Librarian, 25,* 187–200.

Cook, B. (Ed.). (1992). *The electronic journal: The future of serials-based information.* New York: Haworth Press.

Crawford, W., & Gorman, M. (1995). *Future libraries: Dreams, madness & reality.* Chicago: American Library Association.

Eldredge, J. D. (1993). Accuracy of indexing coverage information as reported by serials sources. *Bulletin of the Medical Library Association, 81,* 364–370.

Fortney, L. M., & Basile, V. A. (1996). *Index Medicus price study, 1992–1996.* Birmingham, AL: Ebsco.

Hawbaker, A. C., & Wagner C. K. (1996). Periodical ownership versus full-text online access: A cost-benefit analysis. *Journal of Academic Librarianship, 22,* 105–109.

Reed, K. L. (1995). Citation analysis of faculty publication: Beyond "Science Citation Index" and "Social Sciences Citation Index." *Bulletin of the Medical Library Association, 83,* 503–508.

Tyler, J. K., & Switzer, J. H. (1991). Meeting the information needs of nursing students. *Medical Reference Services Quarterly, 10,* 39–44.

Wood, R. J. (1996). The Conspectus: A collection analysis and development success. *Library Acquisitions: Practice & Theory, 20,* 439–453.

Jonathan DeForest Eldredge

APPENDIX A
DIRECTORIES SPECIFIC TO
COLLECTION DEVELOPMENT*

The Serials Directory
Ebsco Publishing
10 Estes Street
P.O. Box 682
Ipswich, MA 01938–0682

Publishers, Distributors and
Wholesalers of the United States
RR Bowker
121 Chanlon Road
New Providence, NJ 07974

Ulrich's International
Directory of Serials
RR Bowker
121 Chanlon Road
New Providence, NJ 07974

Books in Print
RR Bowker
121 Chanlon Road
New Providence, NJ 07974

APPENDIX B
SAMPLE EVALUATION FORM FOR JOURNALS

EVALUATION BY FACULTY
Possible New Journal Subscription

Journal Title _____

Price $ _____

Please rank this journal according to the following criteria:

	Excellent			*Poor*
1. Expertise of authors	1	2	3	4
2. Importance of topics covered	1	2	3	4
3. Quality of research reported	1	2	3	4
4. Evidence of peer review	1	2	3	4
5. Usefulness to audience(s)	1	2	3	4

---

* Many of the publications are available in public libraries or libraries that are members of the NN/LM, discussed in Chapter 10.

		Excellent			*Poor*
6.	Relevance to organizational program	1	2	3	4
	a. Research				
	b. Clinical Service				
	c. Teaching				
7.	Timeliness of information	1	2	3	4
8.	Usefulness in comparison to other journals covering same subject areas(s)	1	2	3	4

Comments:

Rank the relative strengths of this journal by assigning a number between 1 and 6, but use each number only once:

_____ Expertise of authors

_____ Importance of topics covered

_____ Quality of research reported

_____ Usefulness to audience

_____ Relevance to organizational program

_____ Timeliness of information

9. If you had to substitute this journal for an existing library subscription in the same subject area, which title would you cancel?

Comments:

Your Name: _____

Thank you. Please return to *[name of librarian, name of library]*.

181

Jonathan DeForest Eldredge

APPENDIX C
NURSING ORGANIZATIONS THAT PUBLISH
(ELDREDGE, 1996)

American Academy of Nurse Practitioners

American Association for the History of Nursing

American Association of Colleges of Nursing

American Association of Critical-Care Nurses

American Association of Nurse Anesthetists

American Association of Spinal Cord Injury Nurses

American College of Nurse-Midwives

American Nephrology Nurses' Association

American Organization of Nurse Executives

Association of Operating Room Nurses (AORN)

Association of Women's Health, Obstetric, and Neonatal Nurses (AWHONN)

Canadian Nurses Association

Emergency Nurses Association

International Council of Nurses

National Alliance of Nurse Practitioners

National Association of Orthopaedic Nurses

National Association of Pediatric Nurse Associates and Practitioners

National Council of State Boards of Nursing

National Nurses Society on Addictions

National Organization of Nurse Practitioner Faculty

National Federation for Specialty Nursing Organizations (NFSNO)

6

Cataloging and Processing

Sharon R. Willis, MLS
Margaret M. Jarrette, MLS

The purpose of cataloging and processing materials is to facilitate access and usage. This chapter provides an overview of issues relating to the processing and cataloging of materials for library collections and information centers.

Although numerous sources of ready-to-use cataloging records are available, librarians should be knowledgeable about the authoritative rules and standards governing descriptive cataloging for effective library management. A knowledge of the cataloging process will also enable the librarian to negotiate and judge the quality of information offered by the various vendors of cataloging services, and to develop cataloging records for items when cataloging copy is not available.

CATALOGS AND ACCESS

A record of the holdings in the library or information center should be maintained to provide access to materials. This record is usually a library catalog of some type that provides a record of materials in the collection and their location, and assembles records of materials on the same or related subjects, or by the same authors. Access is provided to items in a collection through names and titles associated with them on the catalog record, as well as through adequate subject analysis and classification. Regardless of the type of catalog (the more common types are the card, online, book, or microform), it should be flexible, allowing for the addition of entries for new acquisitions and removal of records of items withdrawn from the collection; it should be kept up to date, and be accessible to users and staff.

The Card Catalog

Although automation in the library field has greatly increased, the card catalog is still used in many small nursing libraries and information centers as a source for accessing collections. Subject access in a card catalog is necessarily limited, but it allows endless intercalations. From a management point of view, however, cataloging copy for nursing titles and software for catalog cards is readily available from CATLINE, AVLINE, and from some publishers and vendors. Additional information on the card catalog is included in Chapter 4.

The Online Catalog

The online catalog, commonly referred to as an online public access catalog (OPAC), is now considered necessary for libraries with large collections to facilitate ready access to materials in the collection and to enable timely and effective maintenance of cataloging records. The online catalog provides users multiple access points for searching and retrieving information on the status of materials in the collection; authority control over names, series and subjects; and depending upon facilities, can afford access to multiple users from multiple sites.

Usually, online cataloging records are in MARC (MAchine Readable Cataloging) format. This affords the library the option of using available MARC-based services for processing records, producing lists, generating statistics, providing access to materials, and for participating in the sharing of resources. The MARC format, a guide to the data on the catalog record, facilitates computer interpretation of information on a cataloging record and allows the cataloger to manipulate the data when examining, adding, or editing records. The cataloging record is a bibliographic record in MARC format (Figure 6.1) or card format (Figure 6.2), which shows the description of an item; that is, the classification number or call number, the main entry, added entries, subject headings, and added information.

The Library of Congress introduced format integration, a single bibliographic format, to simplify cataloging and informational display for all types of materials. Format integration maintains data elements that can be used to describe many forms of materials—books, serials, visual materials, computer files, maps, music, and so on. Each bibliographic record in the MARC bibliographic format is divided into fields—author, title, publication data, physical description, notes, subject headings, and others. Each field is

010	Library of Congress Control Number (LCCN)
020	International Standard Book Number (ISBN)
050	LC Call Number
060	NLM Call Number
IXX	Main Entry
245	Title Statement
250	Edition Statement
260	Publication Information
300	Physical Description or Collation
4XX	Series Statement
5XX	Notes
6XX	Subject Added Entries
7XX	Added Entries
8XX	Series Added Entries
9XX	Local-use fields

Figure 6.1 Bibliographic Record (MARC Format)

Sharon R. Willis & Margaret M. Jarrette

Call   Main Entry
No.   [Uniform title]
     Title and Statement of Responsibility Area—Edition Area—Publi-
cation, Distribution, etc., Area.
     Physical Description Area—(Series Area).
     Note Area.
     Standard Number and Terms of Availability Area.
     1. Subject Heading(s)   I. Added Entry (Entries).

Figure 6.2   Bibliographic Record (Card Format)

identified with a three-digit code or tag, and is further subdivided
into one or more subfields (Crawford, 1989).

Other Catalog Formats

Although the card and online catalogs are the predominant physical formats used in libraries today, two other forms are used to a
lesser degree: the book catalog and the microform catalog. The
book catalog is the older of the two. Microform catalogs, produced either in microfilm or microfiche, became popular with
the development of computer-output microform (COM). Both the
book and microform catalogs are expensive and time-consuming
to cumulate if original records are not machine-readable. The option to producing cumulations is to produce supplements. This,
however, would require the user to search several sequences of the
book or microform catalog for access to all cataloged materials in
the collection.

The Shelflist

The shelflist may be an online file, a card catalog or part card catalog and part online, depending upon the level of conversion, if
previously in all card format. Records in the shelflist are arranged
by call number order exactly as the items in the collection are

186

located on the shelves. The shelflist may be consulted regularly by the library staff to: verify that a potentially new call number is in current use; record the number of copies owned; locate copies of the same item; use as a control for inventory; and compare subject headings chosen for new materials with those already used for materials having the same or similar classification numbers. It is generally not accessible to the public.

For security—in case of fire, theft, or vandalism—a record of the library's holdings should be stored on microfilm, in machine-readable or other format at a site separate from the library and the card or online catalog.

RETROSPECTIVE CONVERSION

Automation has forced libraries to make a choice: to continue some manual procedures, techniques, and services or to adopt automation. When a library decides to automate, the question is how to handle the old records: Should the library continue to rely on the manual card catalog to access older materials? Should the older records be included in the new system?

Retrospective conversion involves changing a library's catalog cards to electronic format, and this may be done in-house or by vendors. The Online Computer Library Center, Inc. (OCLC) provides guidelines for planning and implementation of retrospective conversion (Online Computer Library Center, Inc., 1988). The library manager needs to:

1. Define its objectives; for example, to change records to AACR2R (Anglo-American Cataloging Rules, second edition, revised) format, reclassify the collection, and so on.

2. Establish a conversion basis, which should be the cataloging source that has the most accurate and complete bibliographic information.

3. Prioritize the conversion project according to available funding.

4. Inventory the collection to determine whether each record is worth converting.

5. Examine the catalog cards to verify that enough information is present to establish a match in a bibliographic utility.

6. Determine the kind of match acceptable to the library.

7. Document the project with clearly defined procedures, incorporating workflow patterns.

8. Define expectations (p. 21).

CATALOGING SOURCES

Because original cataloging is time consuming and requires skill and knowledge in the application of the specific rules and standards for descriptive cataloging, classification, and subject analysis, the trend is to try to keep the amount of original cataloging at a minimum. Using cataloging copy enables the librarian to make items acquired by the library available to library users sooner. In recent years, there has been a proliferation of sources of cataloging copy for the various types of materials acquired by libraries, some of which are discussed here.

Copy Cataloging

Since libraries acquire many of the same materials, duplication of effort can be avoided by first searching for a catalog record in the National Library of Medicine's online databases CATLINE® (CATalog onLINE) or AVLINE® (AudioVisuals onLINE) or in a bibliographic utility such as OCLC (Online Computer Library Center, Inc.) or RLIN (Research Libraries Information Network). Copy editing or copy cataloging can be done directly on the utility with the item in hand, or the library can download (transfer electronically) records to be edited into the local system. If the library is a participating subscriber to the bibliographic utility being used for copy cataloging, cataloging can be done on the local system and uploaded to the utility. The Internet (a computer communication network) is another way to tap into other libraries' catalogs around the world. Bibliographic records of other libraries can be modified to conform to local practices and policies, especially in the subject heading and classification areas. Most libraries will accept a record cataloged by NLM (National Library of Medicine) and LC (Library of Congress). Paraprofessionals perform copy cataloging in many libraries.

CIP (Cataloging in Publication)

These partial bibliographic records, printed on the verso of the title page of most current American books, are based on prepublication data received from the publisher by the Library of Congress. LC forwards core biomedical titles to the National Library of Medicine to catalog. Although CIP records are available in the MARC format, libraries that have no online capabilities can use this printed data inside the book as a basis for cataloging. The CIP record is printed in card format and contains the names of the author/editors, title, series statement, notes, subject and added entries, LC call number (and NLM when appropriate), Dewey Decimal Call number (DDC), the LC control number, and the ISBN (International Standard Book Number). Although CIP records contain useful information such as the form of headings, classification, and subject headings, it must be used with caution because it is based on preliminary information, which might change when the item is published.

Vendors

Bibliographic records are available to local libraries for downloading and editing through cooperative cataloging via bibliographic utilities. Libraries can order items from vendors already cataloged or may order only sets of cards. Some publishers supply catalog cards and shelf-ready books. MARC tapes and cards can be ordered from LC, OCLC, MARCIVE, Inc., and other vendors marketing similar services. Many of these vendors are listed in *The Librarian's Yellow Pages* included under "Cataloging and Processing Aids" at the end of this chapter.

TYPES OF MATERIALS

Depending upon library policy, the size of the collection, and the content of the collection, the various types of materials acquired by the library may receive different treatment (i.e., cataloged versus uncataloged, classification versus assigned accession numbers, a separate versus integrated shelving, and others). For a more efficient workflow, however, a flowchart should be prepared showing how the various materials are processed, from receiving to circulation. The flowchart may show steps for searching; cataloging; ordering cards; stamping ownership marks; applying security tapes, bar codes, labels, or date-due slips; updating of records; and routing of materials for special treatment or processing. The flowchart should be regularly reviewed and updated.

Monographs

A monograph or book is ". . . an item either complete in one part or complete, or intended to be completed, in a finite number of separate parts . . ." (AACR2R, 1988, p. 620). Monographs may be cataloged originally, cataloged on a bibliographic utility, or cataloged offline using information from the National Library of Medicine or other libraries participating in cooperative cataloging. AACR2R should be followed for cataloging monographs unless local changes are indicated.

Serials

A serial is "a publication in any medium issued in successive parts bearing numeric or chronological designations and intended to be continued indefinitely. Serials include periodicals; newspapers; annuals (reports, yearbooks, etc.); the journals, memoirs, proceedings, transactions, etc. of societies; and numbered monographic series" (AACR2R, 1988, p. 622). The term periodicals is frequently used interchangeably for journals, newspapers, and annuals.

Whether and how serial literature will be shelved are administrative decisions often influenced by the size of the collection and available shelving. Some nursing libraries do not catalog periodicals; rather they are shelved separately from the books in an alphabetical arrangement by title. When serials are cataloged, they may be shelved separately from, or interfiled with, books in call number order.

If serials are cataloged, the usual practice in nursing libraries is to establish records using the title as it appears on the item in hand. Cataloging copy for serials is available in the CATLINE database and national bibliographic utilities. AACR2R should also be consulted if the library elects to catalog serials.

Government Publications

These publications include international, national, state, and municipal publications, which may be monographs, serials, or ephemera in print or microforms. Government materials may be cataloged and integrated into the collection with the same classification system, subject headings, and standard bibliographic description used for other formats of the collection—serials, nonbook materials, and so on. If materials are not cataloged, the Superintendent of Documents Classification System (SuDoc) may be used in grouping, filing, or shelving materials by the issuing agencies. SuDoc makes no provision for filing or shelving by subject. The Government Printing Office (GPO) is the authority for names of government agencies, and is accepted as such by the National Library of Medicine and by the Library of Congress.

Nonbook Materials

The size and location of the nonbook or audiovisual collection and how it will be used, the amount of available shelf space, the utilization of special equipment, and the type and format of materials influence the organization and treatment of nonbook materials. (The processing of materials for clinical simulation laboratories is discussed in Chapter 9.) Nonbook materials may be listed and shelved separately; or they may be partially or fully cataloged with cards integrated into the card catalog, as indicated in Chapter 4, but shelved separately. A separate card or other catalog should be considered for nonbook materials in a large collection when there is no online catalog or the collection is not housed and used in the same area as the general collection. If nonbook materials require a temperature-controlled environment, special packaging, and maintenance, they should not be shelved in the main collection. In determining treatment, the main criteria should be the protection of the materials and facilitating maximum utilization.

Cataloging copy for nonbook or audiovisual materials is available from the NLM in its AVLINE (Audiovisuals Online) database or from other bibliographic utilities. AACR2R provides guidelines for cataloging special materials: sound recordings, motion pictures and video recordings, graphic materials, computer files, and three-dimensional artifacts and realia. Nonbook materials may also be classified in the same system as monographs.

Microforms

Microforms may be reproductions of textual or graphic materials or they may be original publications. Because their use requires special equipment, microforms are usually housed separately from other materials. They may be arranged by classification number, title, or accession number. AACR2R provides guidelines for cataloging microforms.

Unpublished Materials and Ephemera

The cataloging and processing of unpublished materials and ephemera should be considered in relation to their historical value and usefulness to primary library clientele. Those of historical value should be treated as archival materials. Others may be placed in a vertical file or given minimal treatment, for example, accessioned, placed in folders, and then shelved or filed. Chapter 7, Special Collections, provides information on the management of unpublished materials.

Historical and Rare Materials

AACR2R provides guidelines on cataloging historical materials. Cataloging copy for historical materials is available in the CATLINE database and on national bibliographic utilities. For additional information on historical and rare materials, refer to Chapter 7.

CATALOGING PROCESS

When a source for copy cataloging is not available for materials received by the library, the librarian must create original cataloging records from scratch. Pending the creation of full original cataloging of an item, it may be shelved and circulated after minimum cataloging or placed in storage for a short period of time until the research for original cataloging is completed.

The cataloging process consists of three interrelated functions: descriptive cataloging, classification, and subject analysis. Each function is governed by specific rules and standards, which should be maintained at the highest level since the intellectual manipulation of data for each item dictates the accessibility of that item to library clientele. Any deviations from AACR2R standards should be considered carefully to ensure that such deviations continue to provide the same level of access to the collection that the standard rules provide.

A library cataloging manual for documenting local cataloging procedures and policies, including deviations from the standards, should be maintained for day-to-day reference and future use by personnel to ensure consistent application of procedures and policies. Furthermore, a local authority file should be maintained listing locally used names, series, and subject headings and kept completely separate from the bibliographic files.

Authority Control

Authority control is "the process of ensuring that every entry—name, uniform title, series, or subject—that is selected as an access point for the public catalog is unique and does not conflict by being identical with any other entry that is already in the catalog or that may be included at a later date. Uniqueness, standardization, and the linkage are the foundation of authority control" (Clack, 1985, pp. 127–128).

Authority control takes some of the burden off the user; that is, a user can assume that all works relating to a name will be found together, or will at least be connected with cross-references. Users do not have to search under alternate forms of names; for example, full name versus initials or maiden name versus married name (Wynar & Taylor, 1992). The unique and consistent treatment of headings enables catalogers to work more rapidly and consistently since they can rely on a list of forms of entries that have already been approved (Bourdon, 1994).

"Authority work includes the research work and intellectual effort involved in creating and updating authority records" (Tillett, 1989, p. 3). The cataloger should examine not only the title page, but other locations within the item for variant forms of the names, particularly the introduction or the preface, where a named conference may be embedded. In order for a heading to be consistently applied to bibliographic records, the cataloger should search the authority file (and/or bibliographic file) to determine whether the name has been used before, and if so, in what form. If the heading is not already established or has been established in a different form, AACR2R rules governing the related heading should be followed.

Reference works such as biographical directories or encyclopedias are useful in resolving conflicts between names and determining relationships among names. Two reference sources for nursing are *Directory of Nurse Researchers* (Sigma Theta Tau

International, 1993), and *American Nursing, a Biographical Dictionary* (Bullough, Church, & Stein, 1988). In the online environment, authority work is facilitated by such features as downloading (electronically transferring records from another online system to the local system).

Names and Series. Authority records are permanently maintained by a library, manually or online, as a cataloging resource representing designated established names, which include: authority data for the preferred form of heading; consulted sources in which information is found about the heading; variant forms, related headings and their corresponding cross-references; historical, biographical, and other information necessary to distinguish one name from another; and cautionary notes about possible confusion among like names for different people or institutions. There are Name Authority Records (NARs) and Series Authority Records (SARs). NARs include authority records for personal, corporate, conference, uniform title, and geographic name headings for jurisdictions. SARs contain information on whether a series access point is to be made for the series on the bibliographic record; whether the phrase is a true series or series-like phrase; and whether the library will classify the series as a collection and therefore shelve all items in the series together or classify these items separately.

Subject Headings. Assigned subject headings in online and card catalogs, or those used in bibliographic records in libraries, are usually selected from a controlled vocabulary, such as MeSH and LCSH, which will be discussed in more depth later in this chapter. A controlled vocabulary generally consists of single nouns, adjectival, conjunctive, and prepositional phrases, as well as inverted headings and headings with subdivisions. Many have a hierarchical structure and provide related concepts and cross-references. Usually, directions and rules for using the terms or subject concepts that make up the controlled vocabulary are supplied by the developer of the controlled vocabulary.

According to Taylor (1995), controlled vocabulary not only allows for consistency in the application of subject headings, it also assists the user in locating the most precise subject, alerts the user to synonyms or near synonyms, clarifies ambiguous terminology, and links related terms and concepts.

Bibliographic Data

An access point is "a name, term, code, etc. under which a bibliographic record may be searched and identified" (AACR2R, 1988, p. 615). In a manual file, access points are traditionally considered names, titles, or subjects placed at the head of a catalog entry. In an online file, access points can include not only author, title, and series, but also other useful retrieval points such as the ISBN, ISSN, LC number, and more. Access points give the user several options in the retrieval of library materials.

The most productive source for all access points is, first, the chief source (usually the title page) followed by other prominent sources (for example, the title page verso, pages preceding the title page, the cover, and the colophon). The table of contents, introduction, and preface also yield information for determining access points.

The description of an item should include as much information as is necessary to distinguish one item from others, and should include its scope, contents, and bibliographic relationships. The data should be presented as simply and concisely as possible and in the same form and order according to corresponding chapters in AACR2R.

AACR2R prescribes the punctuation between and within the designated areas in accordance with International Standard Bibliographic Description (ISBD), an "international agreed-upon framework for cataloging rules for description, which has established essential items of information that must appear in the entry, the order in which these items will be given, and a system of arbitrary punctuation that must be used" (Maxwell, 1989, p. 9). All information on the bibliographic record can be tailored to fit the needs of the individual nursing library.

Main Entry. The access point or heading under which the bibliographic description is entered in the catalog is called the main entry. It is usually the person or body chiefly responsible for the intellectual content of the item in hand. If no principal responsibility is indicated, the title of the work is usually the main entry. Information for the main entry may be ascertained from the item in hand (the title page, verso of the title page, the cover, colophon, etc.) or from an outside source.

Title Entry. The official title for an item is called the title proper, and is generally found on or in the item itself. This title will be used in all library records, in trade catalogs, and in bibliographies to describe a particular item to distinguish it from all others. It may or may not describe the contents of the item. Title main entries include edited works, works with more than three authors or work of unknown authors, sacred scripture works, most serials, and most nonbook materials. A uniform title is chosen when a work has appeared under varying titles. The subtitle or secondary title is often used to expand or limit the title proper. An alternative title is a form of subtitle usually introduced by "or." The parallel title is written in another language or in another script. The cataloger should be alert for spine titles, running titles, or cover titles for which the user may search in the catalog.

Statement of Responsibility. A statement relating to the person or body responsible for the intellectual or artistic contents of a work.

General Material Designation. The general material designation (GMD) is a generic term that identifies the general categories of materials to which an item belongs, and to distinguish one general category from another in a catalog that contains records for more than one type of material—computer files, kits, slides, others. A list of established general material designations is included in AACR2R.

Edition. The edition statement is usually found on the title page, on the verso of the title page, or in the preface, or other front matter. It differs from a printing in that it indicates that changes such as additions, deletions, or modifications have been made from the earlier versions of the item. A printing or reprinting means that more copies of an item were manufactured without changes to supply the demand for the item.

Imprint. The imprint includes the place of publication, the name of the publisher, the date of publication or the place of printing (if the publisher is not known), and the name of the printer (if the name of the publisher is not known).

Collation. The physical description of an item includes the number of pages of a one-volume work or the number of volumes (and/or pages), information about the illustrations, size, and accompanying materials. This area varies with the format of non-book materials.

Series. The series title, an access point, indicates the series to which the book or item belongs, which may be written by one author or several authors on a specific subject commissioned by a publisher, whereby a monographic series title is issued regularly or irregularly, and if numbered, usually in chronological order.

Notes. The notes include information necessary to describe the item in hand that cannot be incorporated in other parts of the record. The notes should be brief, clear, factual, and nonjudgmental.

Subject Headings. Subject access enables a user to locate an item on a known subject, in addition to identifying what the library owns on a given subject. The cataloger may consult the preface, the introduction, foreword, the table of contents, index, bibliographies, and dust jacket in determining the subject content of the item in hand. Subjects are assigned to each item cataloged to reflect the contents as accurately as possible at the level of specificity and terminology most familiar for the library's users.

Once a policy on the use of headings and subheadings has been established, it should be documented and practiced consistently. A local subject authority file is recommended to list locally used subject headings. Cross-references are also important when subject headings have been changed, if a card catalog is still in use. Many libraries place a copy of the current Medical Subject Headings (MeSH®) or Library of Congress Subject Headings (LCSH) near the card catalog so that the printed cross-references may be used. The annual edition of MeSH should be checked for headings that have been added, changed, or deleted. The quarterly edition of the *Library of Congress Cataloging Service Bulletin* should also be checked for subject headings that have been added, changed, or deleted. Additionally, if changes are made as designated by MeSH or the *LC Cataloging Service Bulletin,* a cross-reference card should be inserted to direct the user to the new headings.

Added Entries. Access points other than the main entry are added entries, which provide additional access to materials other than the main entry; for example., coauthors, editors, illustrators, translators, collaborators, previous titles, authors of earlier editions, series or corporate names, subtitles, and others.

Call Number. The call number is the shelf location of an item. Its main three parts are the classification number, the book number, and the date of publication or conference date. Call numbers facilitate the shelving of materials on the same subject together. NLM and LC schedules have useful notes and directions for assigning classification numbers.

Classification numbers obtained from cataloging copy should be examined closely for conformity to local applications prior to acceptance or modification. Appropriate classification is essential for optimal access to items in the collection. The main entry is represented by the book or cutter number. It enables the alphabetical arrangement of authors or titles within the subject area of the classification number.

The *Cutter-Sanborn Three-Figure Author Table* (1969) is used to assign three-digit book numbers representing the first major word of the main entry. Adding a work-mark or a letter from the first major word of the title, in addition to the first three letters of the author's surname will increase specificity. The edition number may also be added after the work-mark to aid in chronological shelving.

The book numbering system of the Library of Congress may be adopted for use in the nursing library.

Another part of the call number is the date of publication. It is essential to add this information for materials in a nursing collection because the currency of information in the collection is important. Having the date of publication on material facilitates the weeding of dated materials. If the material represents proceedings of a workshop, conference, or congress, the date of the meeting rather than the date of publication is most often used. Generally, the size of the collection will determine the complexity of the call number.

The shelflist should be consulted prior to assigning a call number to verify that the number is not currently in use; if it is, the number being assigned should be modified to adhere to the shelflisting practices of the library.

Descriptive Cataloging

"Description is that part of the cataloging process concerned with identification of an item and with recording information about the item in a bibliographic record in such a way that the item will be identified exactly and cannot be confused with any other item" (Wynar & Taylor, 1992, p. 43). *Anglo-American Cataloging Rules,* second edition, 1988 revision (AACR2R), is the authoritative source for descriptive cataloging. The Library of Congress periodically issues interpretations of some of these rules for clarification and/or explanation of LC practice, called *Library of Congress Rule Interpretations* (LCRIs) (Hiatt, 1990). The National Library of Medicine generally follows LCRIs but does occasionally issue its own rule interpretations.

Levels of Description. According to AACR2R (Maxwell, 1989, p. 11), there are three levels of detail in cataloging description. The choice of the level of description by an individual library depends largely on the needs of the library's users and the goals of the library. Different levels may be used by the same library for different materials or due to special circumstances; for example, the first level may be used temporarily to eliminate a backlog. Additionally, libraries using a bibliographic utility may be required to accept a specific national standard for consistency. Each library determines the bibliographic data to include on its records based on its standards, which should allow for local flexibility. Minimum standards should be maintained to accommodate cooperative use of other cataloging records and to allow the merging of other library records into the databases. Since the rules governing the choice of access points and the forms of headings remain the same regardless of the level of description chosen, records created at different levels may be integrated in a single catalog.

The first level of brief cataloging is sufficient to identify materials in small library collections and conform to AACR2R standards:

Title proper.

First statement of responsibility (if different from the main entry heading or if there is no main entry heading).

Edition statement.

Material (or type of publication) details.

First publisher and date of publication.

Pagination.

Note.

Standard book number.

The second level of description, considered a full descriptive record, may be used in medium-sized libraries; it includes:

Title proper.

General material designation (GMD) for nonbook materials.

Parallel title and other title information.

Edition statement.

First statement of responsibility relating to the edition.

Material (or type of publication) details.

First place of publication.

First publisher, date of publication.

Physical description (pagination or number of volumes, illustrative materials and size).

Series statement.

Notes.

Standard number.

The third level of description is appropriate for large libraries and should include all the bibliographic data applicable to the item being cataloged.

The cataloging description level is divided into eight "areas," or major sections, namely:

1. Title and statement of responsibility.
2. Edition.
3. Material (or type of publication) details.
4. Publication, distribution, and so on.
5. Physical description.
6. Series.
7. Note.
8. Standard number and terms of availability.

The order and names of the areas were assigned by the International Standard Bibliographic Description (ISBD), upon which AACR2R is based. Punctuation between and within the areas is clearly defined. Chief sources and prominent sources to be consulted for obtaining information to input into these areas are spelled out in each chapter of AACR2R. Any information not taken from the item being cataloged should be bracketed.

Subject Analysis

Subject headings serve as additional access points to items in a collection. All materials cataloged in a library are not necessarily assigned subject headings nor do they receive full subject analysis. Library policy influences the assigning of subject headings. Current materials on core subjects collected by the library generally receive full-subject analysis. Foreign language materials and/or older materials tend to receive limited or no subject analysis. More general subject headings are assigned to serial publications because of the broadness of their scope. Form subdivisions are generally applied to both serial (e.g., periodicals) and nonprint (e.g., videocassettes) materials.

In assigning subject headings, the most important decision is determining how specific headings should be. Subject headings should never be assigned based on the title alone, because titles can sometimes be misleading. The rule of thumb is that subject headings are assigned only for topics that comprise at least 20 percent of the work (Library of Congress, 1996). Historically, the point is to "summarize the contents of a work rather than provide indexing in depth" (Frantz, 1990, p. 632). Multiple subject headings are usually listed on the bibliographic record in order of importance (primary then secondary). If a single subject heading that adequately describes the content is not available, subheadings or subdivisions are commonly used to achieve specificity; for example, topical, geographic, form, language, topic of the item being cataloged. More than one main heading can be used. The maximum number of subject headings assigned is generally six, although sometimes up to 10 subject headings and/or chronological subdivisions can be used in conjunction with main headings. For consistency, subject headings used on related works such as editions and translations should be taken into consideration when assigning subject headings.

Medical Subject Headings (MeSH®). MeSH is the National Library of Medicine's controlled vocabulary used in indexing materials for the MEDLARS databases and for cataloging books, journals, documents, and nonprint materials (National Library of Medicine, 1996a). It is a hierarchical system of subject headings arranged in both an alphabetical and a hierarchical structure with each subject heading presented along with its assigned tree number(s) for one or more of the alphabetic trees or categories

203

(National Library of Medicine, 1997a; National Library of Medicine, 1997b). A subject heading may be assigned to more than one of the trees or categories. The MeSH categories are shown in Figure 6.3.

MeSH is available in several formats, and it is updated annually. Published as a part of *Index Medicus,* it has both a hierarchical and an alphabetical listing of subject headings. The printed formats used by catalogers are the *Medical Subject Headings— Annotated Alphabetic List* (National Library of Medicine, 1997a), which includes subject headings, cross-references, geographic headings, non-MeSH terms check tags, tree numbers, and notes for indexers, catalogers, and online searchers; *Medical Subject Headings, Tree Structures, 1997* (National Library of Medicine, 1997b), which includes annotations preceding each subcategory in the hierarchical listing of the trees or categories of subject headings that show the relationships between broader and narrower subject headings; the *Permuted Medical Subject Headings, 1997*

A   Anatomy
B   Organisms
C   Diseases
D   Chemicals and Drugs
E   Analytical, Diagnostic, and Therapeutic Techniques and
        Equipment
F   Psychiatry and Psychology
G   Biological Sciences
H   Physical Sciences
I   Anthropology, Education, Sociology, and Social Phenomena
J   Technology, Industry, Agriculture
K   Humanities
L   Information Science
M   Named Groups
N   Health Care
Z   Geographicals

Figure 6.3   MeSH Categories

(National Library of Medicine, 1997d), which includes a display of each MeSH term, cross-references and check tags; and the *Medical Subject Headings—Supplementary Chemical Records, 1997* (National Library of Medicine, 1997c), which includes chemicals mentioned in journals indexed in MEDLINE.

The online version of MeSH used by catalogers is called the MeSH Vocabulary File (sometimes called File MeSH by catalogers), which includes current subject headings, subheadings, and supplementary chemical terms.

Nursing is only one of the many health care fields that MeSH covers. Although MeSH does not have a category exclusively devoted to nursing, a significant number of nursing concepts are represented by subject headings in the M and N categories. According to Brenner and McKinnin (1989, p. 366), however, "seventy percent of CINAHL's controlled vocabulary is identical to the National Library of Medicine's MeSH." This in spite of the fact that a primary focus of CINAHL *(Cumulative Index to Nursing & Allied Health Literature)* is nursing. As the field of nursing changes and becomes more specialized, the MeSH vocabulary is updated annually by subject specialists with input from catalogers, indexers, reference librarians, and health care professionals. MeSH not only has numerous main headings dealing with nursing, but it also has two subheadings exclusively on nursing. /*nursing* and /*nurses' instruction* (National Library of Medicine, 1995).

Library of Congress Subject Headings (LCSH). Library of Congress Subject Headings have been developed in close connection with the LC's collection rather than as a comprehensive system with a structured hierarchical scheme as is the case with MeSH. Similar to MeSH though, LCSH is comprised of main headings and subdivisions. The main headings range from single nouns to complex descriptive phrases. Broader, narrower, related, and synonymous relationships among headings are indicated. Unlike MeSH, corresponding classification numbers are listed with a large number of the subject headings. Four categories of broad subdivisions are found in LCSH: topical, form, chronological, and geographic. Also, LCSH has free-floating subdivisions, that is, subdivisions that can be applied in specifically defined situations.

LCSH is published annually in printed format. In addition, it is available on microfiche, CD-ROM, and in the MARC authority format. The *Subject Cataloging Manual: Subject Headings* (Library of Congress, Cataloging Policy and Support Office, 1996) is an important tool for accurately applying LCSH.

Some nursing libraries may use LCSH instead of MeSH or in conjunction with MeSH. However, MeSH may be more useful because it is specifically designed for collections in the health sciences.

Classification

Classification serves the purpose of grouping similar material in the collection in order to provide a more cohesive shelf arrangement as well as easier access for library users. A formal ordering of library materials is provided, which is "based upon a classification number assigned to the book, representing the main focus of the work and acting as a subject surrogate" (Losee, 1995, p. 45). Classification is beneficial because it provides subject organization of the library's collection in a logical sequence, from general topics to specific topics. Additionally, it enables the user not only to locate a specific item but adjacent items on the same or related subjects.

A classification system consists of notations or class numbers composed of shorthand symbols or codes that are used in translating the meaning of a specific class, division, or subdivision. The notation also serves as a shelf or file address for the cataloged item (Wynar & Taylor, 1992). Captions, notes, and instructions are also included to facilitate use of the classification system.

The National Library of Medicine Classification System. The National Library of Medicine Classification system has been in existence since 1948 and has undergone several revisions since this time. It is a broad classification, covering the field of medicine and related health sciences, and is suitable for any size collection (National Library of Medicine, 1996b).

The National Library of Medicine Classification is a system of mixed notation, wherein alphabetical letters denote broad subject categories, which are further subdivided by numbers. LC schedules are used to supplement the National Library of Medicine Classification for borderline and nonhealth sciences subjects and for general reference materials. Schedules QS through QZ are used for the preclinical sciences. Body systems are classed individually in schedules WE through WL. Each major medical specialty is classified using schedules WM through WW, and W through WZ are used for the health professions and related subjects. Schedules WY covers the nursing materials (National Library of Medicine, 1994).

Within each main schedule, the form numbers 1–49 (or other designated subsections) are used for materials classed for form of presentation (e.g., atlases, dictionaries) or a specific aspect of the subject discussed (e.g., education, legislation). To illustrate this point, *Mosby's Comprehensive Review of Nursing* is classed in the nursing schedule with examination questions as WY 18.2, rather than with the general number WY 100. In general, classification by form takes precedence over classification by subject. The outline of the NLM Classification is shown in Figure 6.4.

The NLM classification is used exclusively in many nursing libraries. The WY schedule (Figure 6.5) was one that required particular attention in the latest revision of the NLM *Classification*. Much needed class numbers were added, such as WY 100.4 for nursing assessment and nursing diagnosis and WY 160.5 for Neurosurgical Nursing. Prior to 1984, background materials on clinical medicine written for nurses were classified in the WY schedule along with materials dealing with nursing procedures in special fields of medicine. Currently, materials on clinical medicine written for nurses are classed with the subject, just as background materials written for other health professionals are classed by subject. The subject headings for these items will generally include the form subheading *nurses' instruction*. Materials about nursing techniques in a special field of medicine or nursing care for a specific disease are classed in the WY schedule. Subject headings for these items will generally include the topical subheading *nursing*.

QS	Human Anatomy	WF	Respiratory System
QT	Physiology	WG	Cardiovascular System
QU	Biochemistry	WH	Hemic and Lymphatic
QV	Pharmacology		Systems
QW	Microbiology and	WI	Digestive System
	Immunology	WJ	Urogenital System
QX	Parasitology	WK	Endocrine System
QY	Clinical Pathology	WL	Nervous System
QZ	Pathology	WM	Psychiatry
W	Health Professions	WN	Radiology. Diagnostic
WA	Public Health		Imaging
WB	Practice of Medicine	WO	Surgery
WC	Communicable	WP	Gynecology
	Diseases	WQ	Obstetrics
WD 100	Nutrition Disorders	WR	Dermatology
WD 200	Metabolic Diseases	WS	Pediatrics
WD 300	Immunologic and	WT	Geriatrics. Chronic
	Collagen Diseases.		Disease
	Hypersensitivity	WU	Dentistry. Oral Surgery
WD 400	Animal Poisons	WV	Otolaryngology
WD 500	Plant Poisons	WW	Ophthalmology
WD 600	Diseases and Injuries	WX	Hospital and other Health
	Caused by Physical		Facilities
	Agents	WY	Nursing
WD 700	Aviation and Space	WZ	History of Medicine. 19th
	Medicine		Century Schedule
WE	Musculoskeletal		
	System		

Figure 6.4   Outline of NLM Classification

WY 1–100.5	General
WY 101–145	Special Fields in Nursing
WY 150–164	Nursing Techniques in Special Fields of Medicine
WY 191–200	Other Nursing Services
WY 300	By Country

Figure 6.5   NLM Classification WY Schedule

The Library of Congress Classification System. Beginning in 1899, the Library of Congress Classification system (Figure 6.6) was developed and used as a practical classification for its current and future holdings, based on the relationship of subjects as represented in its collection. As an enumerative system, the 21 main classes are divided into subclasses, which are further subdivided by integral numbers. Class Q (Science) and Class R (Medicine) are the two classes used by some nursing libraries because their order begins with the natural sciences, and includes the preclinical sciences of anatomy and physiology and medicine with its specialties.

The major disadvantage in using the LC classification system for nursing materials is the dispersion of subject materials. Nursing

A	General Works
B	Philosophy, Psychology, Religion
C	Auxiliary Sciences of History
D	History, General and Old World
E-F	History, American
G	Geography, Anthropology, Recreation
H	Social Sciences
J	Political Science
K	Law
L	Education
M	Music and Books on Music
N	Fine Arts
P	Languages and Literature
Q	Science
R	Medicine
S	Agriculture
T	Technology
U	Military Science
V	Naval Science
Z	Bibliography, Library Science

Figure 6.6 Outline of the Library of Congress Classification

209

materials are in the RT class and scattered throughout the other subdivisions of the schedule. Also, the numbers in the LC system tend to be more complex and longer. Still, some nursing libraries have been able to adapt the LC Classification for classifying their materials.

The Dewey Decimal Classification System. All knowledge is represented in the Dewy Decimal Classification System by 10 broad classes, as shown in Figure 6.7. It is a philosophical system that uses the decimal principle and mnemonic devices. The structure is hierarchical. Each broad class is divided into 10 divisions, each of which may have 10 sections, which may be further subdivided decimally. The classification develops progressively from the general to the specific in disciplinary and subject relationships. Although some nursing schools have been able to adapt the Dewey Decimal Classification System for use, it is not recommended for cataloging nursing literature because of its general subdivisions and notation.

Other Classification Systems. The majority of nursing libraries use either the NLM or LC Classification systems, or a combination of both. Other libraries use a form of in-house classification system. If a nursing school has materials cataloged using

000	Generalities
100	Philosophy and Psychology
200	Religion
300	Social Sciences
400	Language
500	Natural Sciences and Mathematics
600	Technology and Applied Sciences
700	The Arts
800	Literature and Rhetoric
900	Geography and History

Figure 6.7   Classes of the Dewey Decimal Classification System

the Boston Medical Library Classification, the Cunningham Classification, or the Bellevue Classification System as referred to by Scheerer and Hines (1974), and a change to another system is planned, it would probably be more economical to leave older materials as they are and to begin classifying current materials using the NLM or LC classification systems. This will enable the library to take advantage of the various sources of cataloging copy and to participate in cooperative cataloging ventures.

INTEGRATED SYSTEMS

Libraries today are selecting online systems that will provide users with the most effective and efficient service possible. Integrated Library Systems (ILS) allow the same bibliographic data describing library materials to be accessed through many modules; for example, acquisitions, cataloging, interlibrary loan, public catalog, and circulation. The user searches one master database rather than several different modules. In making a selection, libraries may choose systems different from those used by other libraries in similar environments. Factors to consider are: flexibility; efficient system functionality, adherence to library and computing/communication standards, stability and dependability, and reasonable cost. Vendors of integrated library systems may be found in *The Librarians' Yellow Pages* given in the "Cataloging and Processing Aids" at the end of this chapter. Some of the most widely used integrated systems include DRA (Data Research Associates), Horizon, NOTIS System, Dynix, VTLS, and Unicorn System by SIRSI Corp.

COOPERATIVE CATALOGING AND ONLINE SYSTEMS

The prevalence and use of automated bibliographic databases have created an entirely new and different approach to the management of cataloging materials. Consequently, materials get on the shelves faster, the catalogers spend less time on routine procedures and more time on original cataloging and research, and the cost of

211

cataloging an item is contained. The development of MARC has greatly facilitated cooperative cataloging via bibliographic utilities. Participation in national cooperative programs and projects offer significant benefits to participants.

Bibliographic Utilities

Online Computer Library Center (OCLC). OCLC, the oldest of the bibliographic utilities, and online since 1971, is a nonprofit membership organization that is widely used in the United States. In addition to online and CD-ROM products, and card production, it provides services for retrospective conversion, cataloging, interlibrary loan, collection development, bibliographic verification, and reference searching. The database consists of LC MARC tapes, NLM's CATLINE tapes, CONSER (Conversion of Serials) and records contributed by its participants.

Subsystems available to subscribers are: interlibrary loan, serials control and union listing, and acquisitions. Smaller libraries may join by a dial-up telephone connection to OCLC, or join a cluster or small consortium in an area where cooperative cataloging and processing services are provided by larger libraries. Medium-sized nursing libraries, whether affiliated with a main university that uses OCLC or larger hospital libraries, may find it beneficial to have their own OCLC membership and terminals for cataloging, interlibrary loan, serials control, acquisitions, and reference.

Research Libraries Information Network (RLIN). RLIN is an automated network of the Research Libraries Group (RLG). RLG operates four independent but interrelated programs: RLIN, shared resources, collection management and development, and preservation. RLIN is a resource-sharing network for its members; its subsystems are acquisitions and interlibrary loan. The database consists of LC MARC tapes for books, maps, serials, sound recordings, scores, audiovisual materials, and computer files; NLM's CATLINE tapes; CONSER records and records of participating libraries.

212

Western Library Network (WLN). WLN is a resource-sharing network that began operating in 1976 for the state of Washington and to provide a multistate computer service for other libraries. The WLN database consists of LC MARC tapes, LC Authority Files, and records of the participating libraries. Its three subsystems are bibliographic, batch retrospective conversion, and acquisitions. Products provided include COM masters on fiche, film, or paper; catalog cards, labels; and printed bibliographies.

NLM Sources. The Cataloging Section of the NLM produces two machine readable databases that are a part of the Library's computer-based Medical Literature Analysis and Retrieval System (MEDLARS): CATLINE (CATalog onLINE), which contains bibliographic records created by NLM catalogers for incunabula and printed books and serials published since the fifteenth century; AVLINE (AudioVisuals onLINE), which contains bibliographic records for nonprint materials in a variety of formats such as video-cassettes, audiocassettes, 16mm films, filmstrips and slides, computer software, videodiscs, CD-ROMS, and more. These databases are available directly from the NLM via the MEDLARS connection or through the Internet to NLM's online catalog, NLM Locator. CATLINE and AVLINE are available in MARC format on a tape subscription basis.

CONCLUSION

All aspects of cataloging—description of the item, authority control, providing access points, assigning subject analysis and classification—are important to ensure that the user has sufficient information to locate materials in the nursing collection. Libraries are faced with many decision points in the process, including form of catalog to use, how to handle divergent types of materials, and the "best, fastest, cheapest" source of cataloging data. The use of AACR2R and MARC formats has promoted standardization in the cataloging community, and cooperative efforts among libraries via bibliographic utilities has facilitated the cataloging process. Catalogers need to stay abreast of new developments in the field so that appropriate innovations can be implemented in a timely manner.

REFERENCES

Anglo-American cataloging rules (2nd ed., rev.). (1988). Chicago: American Library Association.

Bourdon, F. (1994, June). Name authority control in an international context and the role of the national bibliographic agency (presented at IFLA's UBC/UNIMARC Seminar, Vilnius). *International Cataloguing and Bibliographic Control, 23,* 71–77.

Brenner, S. H., & McKinnin, E. J. (1989). CINAHL and MEDLINE: A comparison of indexing practices. *Bulletin of the Medical Library Association, 77,* 366–371.

Bullough, V. L., Church, O. M., & Stein, A. P. (1988). *American nursing: A biographical dictionary.* New York: Garland.

Cataloging Policy and Support Office. (1996). *Subject cataloging manual. Subject headings* (5th ed.). Washington, DC: Cataloging Distribution Service, Library of Congress.

Clack, D. H. (1985). Authority control: Issues and answers. In *Libraries in the '80s* (pp. 127–140). New York: Haworth Press.

Crawford, W. (1989). *MARC for library use: Understanding Integrated US-MARC* (2nd ed.). Boston: G.K. Hall.

Cutter, C. A. (1969). *Cutter-Sanborn three-figure author table* (rev.) Chicopee, MA: H.R. Huntting.

Frantz, P. (1990). A gaping black hole in the bibliographic universe: In the flurry to explore access frontiers, books have been left out: One librarian has a plan for getting at those chapters lost in space. *American Libraries, 21,* 632–633.

Hiatt, R. M. (1990). *Library of Congress rule interpretations* (2nd ed.). Washington, DC: Cataloging Distribution Service, Library of Congress.

Losee, R. M. (1995). How to study classification systems and their appropriateness for individual institutions. *Cataloging & Classification Quarterly, 19,* 45–58.

Maxwell, M. F. (1989). *Handbook for AACR2 1988 revision: Explaining and illustrating the Anglo-American cataloging rules.* Chicago: American Library Association.

National Library of Medicine. (1994). *National Library of Medicine classification: A scheme for the shelf arrangement of library materials in the field of medicine and its related sciences* (5th ed.). Bethesda, MD: National Library of Medicine.

National Library of Medicine. (1995). *MEDLARS indexing manual*. Bethesda, MD: National Library of Medicine.

National Library of Medicine. (1996a). *Medical subject headings (MeSH®). National Library of Medicine fact sheet*. Bethesda, MD: National Library of Medicine.

National Library of Medicine. (1996b). *NLM classification. National library of medicine fact sheet*. Bethesda, MD: National Library of Medicine.

National Library of Medicine. (1997a). *Medical subject headings, annotated alphabetic list, 1997*. Bethesda, MD: National Library of Medicine.

National Library of Medicine. (1997b). *Medical subject headings, tree structures, 1997*. Bethesda, MD: National Library of Medicine.

National Library of Medicine. (1997c). *Medical subject headings—Supplementary chemical records, 1997*. Bethesda, MD: National Library of Medicine.

National Library of Medicine. (1997d). *Permuted medical subject headings, 1997*. Bethesda, MD: National Library of Medicine.

Online Computer Library Center, Inc. (1988). Retrospective conversion: Guidelines for libraries. *Information Reports & Bibliographies, 17*(5), 21–24.

Scheerer, G., & Hines, L. E. (1974). Classification systems used in medical libraries. *Bulletin of the Medical Library Association, 62,* 273–280.

Sigma Theta Tau International. (1993). *Directory of nurse researchers*. Indianapolis, IN: Sigma Theta Tau, National Honor Society of Nursing.

Taylor, A. G. (1995). On the subject of subjects (controversies in subject cataloging). *The Journal of Academic Librarianship, 21,* 484–491.

Tillett, B. B. (1989). Considerations for authority control in the online environment. In B. B. Tillett (Ed.), *Authority control in the online environment: Considerations and practices* (pp. 1–12). New York: Haworth Press.

Wynar, B., & Taylor, A. G. (Eds.). (1992). *Introduction to cataloging and classification* (8th ed.). Englewood, CO: Libraries Unlimited.

SUGGESTED READINGS

Boss, R. W., & Espo, H. (1987). Standards, database design, & retrospective conversion. *Library Journal, 112*(16), 54–58.

Flannery, M. R. (1995). Cataloging Internet resources. *Bulletin of the Medical Library Association, 83,* 211–215.

Palmer, J. W. (1986). Subject authority control and syndetic structure—myth and realities; an inquiry into certain subject heading practices and some questions about their implications. *Cataloging & Classification Quarterly, 7,* 71–95.

Svenonius, E., & McGarry, D. (1993). Objectivity in evaluating subject heading assignment. *Cataloging & Classification Quarterly, 16,* 5–40.

Sharon R. Willis & Margaret M. Jarrette

CATALOGING AND PROCESSING AIDS

Aluri, R., Kemp, D., Alasdair, B., & John J. (1991). *Subject analysis in online catalogs.* Englewood, CO: Libraries Unlimited.

American Library Association, Filing Committee. (1980). *ALA filing rules.* Chicago: American Library Association.

Anglo-American Cataloging Rules. (2nd ed., rev.). (1988). Chicago: American Library Association.

Byrne, D. J. (1991). *MARC Manual: Understanding and using MARC records.* Englewood, CO: Libraries Unlimited.

Cataloging Policy and Support Office. (1996). *Subject cataloging manual. Subject headings* (5th ed.). Washington, DC: Cataloging Distribution Service, Library of Congress.

Clack, D. H. (1990). *Authority control, principles, applications, and instructions.* Chicago: American Library Association.

Crawford, W. (1989). *MARC for library use: Understanding integrated US-MARC* (2nd ed.). Boston: G.K. Hall.

Cutter, C. A. (1969). *Cutter-Sanborn three-figure author table* (rev.). Chicopee, MA: H.R. Huntting.

Format Integration and Its Effect on the USMARC Bibliographic Format. (1995). Washington, DC: Cataloging Distribution Service, Library of Congress.

Guidelines for Bibliographic Description of Interactive Multimedia. (1994). Chicago: American Library Association.

Hallan, A. (1989). *Cataloging rules for the description of looseleaf publications* (2nd ed.). Washington, DC: Library of Congress.

Hensen, S. L. (1989). *Archives, personal papers, and manuscripts* (2nd ed.). Chicago: Society of American Archivists.

The librarians' yellow pages: Publications, products & services for libraries & information centers. (1997). Larchmont, New York: Garance. (Available from: Garance, Inc., P.O. Box 179, Larchmont, NY 10538; 800-235-9723; Fax: 914-833-3053.)

Library of Congress classification. R. Medicine. (1995). Washington, DC: Library of Congress.

Maxwell, M. F. (1989). *Handbook for AACR2 1988 revision : Explaining and illustrating the Anglo-American cataloging rules.* Chicago: American Library Association.

National Library of Medicine. (1994). *National Library of Medicine classification: A scheme for the shelf arrangement of library materials in the field of medicine and its related sciences* (5th ed.). Bethesda, MD: National Library of Medicine.

National Library of Medicine. (1997). *Medical subject headings, annotated alphabetic list, 1997.* Bethesda, MD: National Library of Medicine.

National Library of Medicine. (1997). *Medical subject headings, tree structures, 1997.* Bethesda, MD: National Library of Medicine.

National Library of Medicine. (1997). *Medical subject headings—Supplementary chemical records, 1997.* Bethesda, MD: National Library of Medicine.

National Library of Medicine. (1997). *Permuted medical subject headings, 1997.* Bethesda, MD: National Library of Medicine.

Olson, N. B. (1988). *Cataloging microcomputer software: A manual to accompany AACR2, chapter 9, computer files.* Englewood, CO: Libraries Unlimited.

Saye, J. D., & Vellucci, S. L. (1989). *Notes in the catalog record: Based on AACR2 and LC interpretations.* Chicago: American Library Association.

Taylor, A. G. (1988). *Cataloging with copy: Decision-maker's handbook* (2nd ed.). Englewood, CO: Libraries Unlimited.

Weihs, J. (1991). *The integrated library: Encouraging access to multimedia materials* (3rd ed.). Ottawa: Canadian Library Association.

Wynar, B., & Taylor, A. G. (1992). *Introduction to cataloging and classification* (8th ed.). Englewood, CO: Libraries Unlimited.

7

Special Collections

Julie M. Pavri, MSN, MLS

While current monographs and serials typically constitute the bulk of nursing library holdings, other materials frequently are forwarded to the library for "safekeeping." Organizational records, photographs, personal papers, old audiovisual materials and books, and even artifacts such as uniforms, caps, and nursing pins may find their way into the nursing library. For administrative convenience, these miscellaneous nontraditional library materials are often grouped under the heading of "special collections," which, for the purposes of this chapter, will refer to archives, manuscript collections, artifacts, and rare books. Although these terms are often used interchangeably, *archives* is used here to refer to the noncurrent records of an institution or organization that have been selected for preservation because of their enduring value, while *manuscript collections* refers to the personal papers of an individual or an artificial collection of materials from various sources. All of these materials require special handling because of their uniqueness, rarity, or format.

Unlike most library materials, which are published, archives and manuscript collections are unique. In most cases, it is unlikely that copies or duplicates exist. Therefore, care must be taken to preserve the materials, and library classification systems need to be replaced by more thorough descriptive practices in order in ensure access. Ephemera or old books may not be unique, but because of their rarity require careful handling and preservation measures. All special collections materials require additional security procedures and a controlled environment. Indeed, in order to ensure the preservation and accessibility for research of these materials, a well-designed program is imperative. This chapter provides a broad overview of the basic components of a special collections program; it is designed to introduce the topic rather than to give step-by-step instructions. The reference list includes resources that provide detailed information and guidance on each of the topics addressed.

ESTABLISHING A SPECIAL COLLECTIONS PROGRAM

Inventory and Evaluation

The first step in establishing a special collections program is to conduct an inventory and evaluation process. This involves identifying and listing all special collections materials currently held or proposed for inclusion. The quantity, type, age, and condition of the materials should be noted. This inventory forms the basis of the evaluation process to determine the best disposition plan for the materials.

The decision to develop a special collections program must be based on the careful consideration of many factors. As part of the deliberation process, it is helpful to visit other libraries with established special collections programs as well as archives and manuscript repositories. Because the nature of archival work differs from that of libraries, this is especially important if staff have not had previous experience in historical records programs. Once the full scope of the project has been considered, the decision can be made to establish the program or deposit the materials elsewhere. It is imperative that this decision be based on the determination of the *best* way to preserve and to make available for research the materials under consideration. The following questions should be posed and considered as part of this process.

Does a special collections program fit into the mission of the library or parent institution? The goals and/or mission statement must be thoroughly examined to determine how a special collections program would fit into the overall library or institutional program. If there is a strong commitment to the preservation and on-site maintenance of the materials, it may be appropriate to alter the goals or mission to assure that there is a clear understanding of how the program fits into the total program, and to verify that administrative and financial supports are in place, which are necessary to provide a quality program. A library that supports a school of nursing with a strong history component might choose to develop special collections rich in rare books and manuscript collections. A hospital library may include the hospital archives and personal papers of staff members in its holdings.

Does the special collections program support the scope of the library holdings? Special collections that augment current holdings enhance the value of the total library program. For instance, archives and manuscript collections can provide primary source materials that add depth to an existing historical monograph collection.

Are resources available to establish and maintain a program? The development of an historical records program requires an on-going and long-term commitment of the parent institution or organization to support, preserve, and make available a unique group of historical materials. Institutional commitment must include long-term financial resources and a willingness to give the program the necessary authority to carry out its mission. Financial considerations must include start-up costs as well as ongoing expenses. Current space allocation must be examined to determine whether construction or renovation will be necessary. Necessary equipment, such as shelving and computers must be identified, as well as supplies required for start-up. Ongoing expenses include supplies and office maintenance, such as postage, telephone service, and staff expenses. The expectation that existing staff can absorb the additional workload must be supported by a realistic estimate of the time and expense required to receive additional training, provide ongoing staff development, and maintain the special collections materials. Consultants may need to be hired to provide expertise in start-up procedures. Staff should have at least a strong interest in history (Yakel, 1994). It is important to recognize that an historical records program differs significantly from a library, and a librarian with no archival training will need to attend workshops and training programs to become thoroughly familiar with archival practices.

If necessary, outside funding sources may need to be identified to provide materials, make environmental modifications, and supply personnel. Local, state, and federal programs may provide grants to cover some costs. Volunteer organizations may be formed to raise funds; or existing groups such as alumni associations may be enlisted to provide additional program support. Special collections programs should not be expected to generate revenue. However, good historical records programs that include institutional archives typically provide administrative research services, which soon become invaluable.

Is there a need for the new collection? Are the materials duplicated elsewhere? Ephemera, audiovisual materials, rare books, and other published materials may already be readily available elsewhere, thus the resources might be better directed to other areas. Contact other repositories to determine how a new special collections program would fit into a wider nursing or health care documentation plan. Cooperative efforts between libraries can reduce duplication and provide broader overall access to historical materials. Has a documentation strategy been developed that might include your institution? Such strategies place individual repositories into the larger context of the documentation universe of a specified issue, activity, or geographic area. Institutional planning can then be based on the larger strategy. Understanding the larger context, the individual repository can subsequently identify specific areas to document. Such planning reduces duplicative efforts while assuring the most comprehensive documentation. Although nursing has no national documentation plan, there may be local or regional documentation strategies that would be applicable to your institution.

Is the library the most appropriate repository for the materials? Many materials that make their way to the library clearly have a strong association. Organizational records and old books, audiovisual materials, and ephemera from the parent institution have a "natural home" within that institution's library. Materials without these strong ties may be better placed elsewhere.

Deposit of Materials

The decision not to set up a program may be more difficult than establishing an inadequate program (Yakel, 1994). If, after careful consideration, it is determined that materials should be deposited elsewhere, possible repositories must be considered. Preferably historical collections will be preserved closest to their "natural home." The natural home of the records of a closed school of nursing might be the archives or historical collection of the hospital or college that sponsored the program. If there is no hospital or college archives, the local or state historical society might be an option. The manuscript collection of an individual nurse might be deposited in the archives of his or her alma mater or of the hospital at which he or she practiced for most of his or her career. Nursing records often are undervalued, so it is important that a repository that places a clear value on historical nursing materials be selected. Placement of materials in a good repository should be viewed as the best way of preserving the heritage, not "giving away or losing one's history" (Yakel, 1994, p. 8). When looking for a repository, look at the organization's ability to organize, maintain, and provide access to records. Be aware of the costs of such programs. There may be a one-time or an annual fee. Investigate all policies, and make certain that any restrictions or special instructions are clearly specified in writing as part of the deed of gift or certificate of deposit. Responsibilities of both the donor and the repository should be clearly stated (Yakel, 1994, p. 12).

Organizations That Accept Nursing Materials

A wide variety of institutions and organizations may have formal archives programs that maintain and preserve historical nursing materials:

Julie M. Pavri

- Local historical societies and libraries may have personal and family papers and artifacts of local nurses.

- Hospitals, colleges, and universities, either formally or informally, may maintain the archives, as well as related manuscript and archival collections, of the institution. Thus, a hospital archives program might maintain the hospital's archives as well as the records of the affiliated medical school and school of nursing, plus the personal papers of former staff.

- Some colleges and universities maintain specialized collections that may include nursing records. The Women's Archives at Radcliffe College, for instance, maintain nursing records among its collections.

- Local, state, and federal governments may maintain nursing records. The state archives may preserve the records of the State Board for Nursing or the Department of Health. National repositories such as the National Archives and the History of Medicine Division of the National Library of Medicine maintain nursing records as well.

- Many specialized repositories, such as the archives of religious orders, contain nursing materials, and many museums include nursing artifacts among their holdings.

- A few repositories are devoted exclusively to historical nursing materials. The Nutting Collection and the Nursing Archives are two collections of nursing materials that are national in scope. In addition, a small number of regional centers are focused on the collection and use of historical nursing materials.

The Nutting Collection housed in the Special Collections area of the Milbank Library, Teachers College, Columbia University, was established in 1920, and continues today as the premier collection of historical nursing materials. In addition to this extensive collection of monographs and other publications, this repository maintains the archives of Teachers College, including the Nursing

Education Department, the alumni associations, and other organizations and individuals with a strong relationship to the college. The archival collections include the meticulously maintained records of Teachers College's hospital economics course, and the papers of Adelaide Nutting, Isabel Stewart, and other nursing leaders. While active collecting of archival materials is limited to the college, the inclusion of the Nutting Collection and the wide influence of the nursing leaders associated with Teachers College makes this repository national in scope.

The second true national nursing repository is the Nursing Archives maintained at Boston University's Mugar Library. In 1966, Boston University agreed to accept the School of Nursing's historical collection and provide space for a nursing archive. This initiative was aided by a grant from the United States Public Health Service in 1967. When the Nursing Archives at Mugar was designated as the official depository of the records of the American Journal of Nursing Company and the American Nurses Association in 1971, it achieved national status. This repository continues to collect and preserve significant items documenting nursing history, including its social role and impact on health and welfare. It has a large collection of institutional and organizational records and the papers and memorabilia of individuals.

Four large regional centers are devoted exclusively to historical nursing collections. In addition to maintaining archives, manuscript collections, artifacts and historical monographs, most of these centers also engage in a variety of activities to promote the history of the profession, such as developing exhibits; publishing newsletters, books, and conference proceedings; awarding scholarships; and sponsoring conferences. Staff at the centers are very knowledgeable and are excellent resources in the search for an appropriate repository for organizational records or personal papers.

The Center for Nursing Historical Inquiry at the University of Virginia Health Sciences Center was established in 1991 to support historical scholarship in nursing and to disseminate findings. This center focuses on the southern region of the United States, and its collections currently include the archives of the

Julie M. Pavri

National Association of Pediatric Nurse Practitioners, the manuscript collections of individual nurses, and an impressive photograph collection.

The Center for the Study of the History of Nursing at the University of Pennsylvania was founded in 1985 to encourage and facilitate historical scholarship on health care history and nursing in the Mid-Atlantic region. It serves as a national center for visiting nurse association collections, and has records of hospitals, health care agencies, nursing schools, and nursing leaders.

The Foundation of the New York State Nurses Association Center for History was established in 1989 to ensure that records documenting the history of the nursing profession in New York state are preserved, understood, and used. The Foundation Center for History maintains several large organizational archives, including the records of the New York State Nurses Association and several of its constituent district nurses associations, the National Student Nurses Association, and Nurses House, as well as manuscript collections of New York nurses.

The Midwest Nursing History Resource Center at the University of Illinois at Chicago opened in 1982 as a repository for historically significant documents relating to nursing history in the Midwest. Holdings include the records of several schools of nursing, the records of various midwest nursing organizations, and manuscript collections of nursing leaders.

Formulating Policies

Once the decision to establish a special collections program has been made, a mission statement should be prepared, defining the repository's purpose and stating its relationship to the parent institution or organization; all other policies will be based on this statement. It should be short and concise, and include the groups, activities, or experiences the program documents; why the program is initiated; what it collects; and whom it serves (Wilsted & Nolte, 1991). Broad, long-range program goals can be established once the mission statement has been prepared and accepted administratively; and from the goals, more specific objectives can be

226

developed. A prioritized list of objectives forms the basis for a work plan and periodic program review and evaluation.

The collecting policy, based on the program's mission statement, is the basis of an acquisitions plan. The collecting policy specifically identifies the types of materials the program accepts into its collections. The policy should be based on available resources, and take into consideration the quality of the documentation, the priorities and limitations of the collection, agreements with other repositories, and the projected user population (McCall & Mis, 1995; Yakel, 1994). Appraisal guidelines may also be formulated to determine whether materials fit into the collecting policy.

COMPONENTS OF A SPECIAL COLLECTIONS PROGRAM

Accessioning

Accessioning is the process of accepting custody of materials, establishing a basic level of understanding of the informational content of the materials *(intellectual control)*, and tracking the physical location of the materials *(physical control)*. Receiving materials, documenting legal transfer of the property, and maintaining ongoing records of the physical location of the materials are components of the accessioning process.

Records Management. If the archives of the parent institution are included in the program's collecting policy, establishment of a records management program may be included within the scope of the special collections program. A records management program identifies the various types of records created or maintained by an institution or organization, and assigns a retention period and method of disposition for each record type.

A thorough inventory of organizational records is the first step in establishing a records management program. The type of record (e.g., correspondence), quantity (linear feet or number of items), inclusive dates, office of origin, frequency of use, format, and other information is recorded and analyzed. Research is conducted to determine any legal and administrative retention requirements before retention periods are established. Typically, some records are deemed temporary and may be discarded after a specified time period, while other records are identified as having enduring value, and hence are scheduled for transfer to the archives at specified intervals. Records that are essential for the operations of the organization are termed *vital records*. These require special security and environmental considerations because of their value to the day-to-day operations of the organization. A records management program organizes the disposition of all the records of an organization. However, only those records designated as worthy of permanent retention and no longer needed in active files would go into an archives or special collections program.

Accession Log. Whether transferred from a records management program, found in a storage area, or donated by an individual, once materials are received into the special collections program, an accession log provides a means for documenting its arrival. The accession is assigned a unique number in the log, along with the date and origin of the materials. Physical location of the materials is entered into the log or into a separate locator system.

Transmittal Documentation. Records transferred to the archives from a records management program are accompanied by a transfer form, which becomes part of the permanent accession record. Deed of gift forms are used to transfer ownership of materials from an individual or organization to the special collections program, while deposit agreements document a deposit that does not transfer ownership. All agreements with donors or depositors should specify any access restrictions to the materials, and address copyright, literary rights, and any legal restrictions. These agreements and transmittal documentation are retained as permanent records in the accession files of the materials received.

Other Accessioning Tasks. As part of the accessioning process, the records are examined, and a basic level of control is established for the collection. After records are examined, they may be placed into standardized containers, in the order in which the records were transferred. Oversized materials and records in nonpaper formats should be moved to more appropriate containers; the removal and the original location should be noted. The physical characteristics of the materials should be detailed, including the physical condition and possible preservation needs. A preliminary listing of the contents of each container should provide a basic level of access to the materials until further processing can be completed. During the accessioning process, information should be recorded on the subject content of the collection and on the organization, office, or individual that created and used the materials (Miller, 1990).

Arrangement and Description

Arrangement of Archival Records. Classification systems guide librarians in the arrangement of library materials. The arrangement of archival and manuscript collections are guided by quite different principles: the principle of provenance and the principle of the sanctity of original order. Provenance refers to the place of origin of the collections. First and foremost, records that were created and maintained by an organization or an individual in the conduct of day-to-day activities must be kept together, and must not be mixed with materials from a different provenance. The second principle states that the order in which the records were actively used must be preserved or reconstructed whenever possible. When both principles are applied in the arrangement of records, valuable information on the context in which the records were created is preserved, thus enhancing the value of the collections. In rare cases, when the original order cannot be discerned, or the materials have clearly been amassed haphazardly, imposing a system of arrangement may be necessary.

The information gathered during the accessioning process forms the basis for a thorough analysis of the research value, preservation needs, and arrangement and description required to provide access to the information contained in the records. The needs and value of each collection must then be determined within the context of the entire scope of the special collections holdings. Next, priorities need to be established, based on the mission, resources, and users of the program (Miller, 1990). These priorities should indicate the order in which collections, or a backlog of collections, are arranged and described, as well as the level of arrangement and description. Resources must be carefully allocated to provide access and to preserve as many of the materials as possible. It is desirable to provide broad access to as many collections as possible, through a rough arrangement and brief, general description. Later, efforts can be directed toward a more thorough arrangement and description of the more significant collections. The goal should be to make as many collections available for research use as quickly as possible. In a new program, this may involve broadly arranging and describing collections to provide initial broad access, followed by scheduling more refined and detailed stages.

The first step in the arrangement of a collection is to build upon the information gathered during accessioning to determine or to verify provenance and to ascertain the original order of the materials. In archives of large organizations, the materials will most likely be grouped according to office or department. Within these broad divisions, the next step is to identify the natural groupings into which the records fall. These natural groupings, typically called *record series,* consist of groups of records brought together during active use, and organized and maintained as a unit because of similarity of format, function, or content. Examples of record series include correspondence, personnel records, photographs, subject files, and so forth. Based on the information gathered, a plan for grouping and ordering the records can be developed.

Archival records and manuscript collections can be arranged broadly by collection or department, by record series, by file unit (folder, volume, etc.), and by item. Arranging each document in a collection is considered to be arrangement at the item level, and can be extremely time-consuming and costly. In most cases, item-level arrangement is an unrealistic goal. Most repositories do not have the luxury of available resources to arrange and describe each collection at the document or even at the file folder level. It is considered essential, however, that materials be arranged and described at the record series level (State Archives and Records Administration, 1988).

Description of Archival Records. Archival description is the process of communicating information about groups of records to potential users, and requires "both historical research skills and techniques from library and information science" (Miller, 1990). Because of the unique nature of archives and manuscript collections, thorough description is essential to provide adequate access. A variety of descriptive techniques called *finding aids* assist the potential researcher in determining whether a group of records has information relevant to the research topic, and assist staff in locating information.

As with arrangement, there are several levels of description. The repository may have a broad guide to its holdings or a brochure that describes in general terms the types of materials available for research. Other finding aids include descriptions of records at the collection and record series levels, accession forms, lists of boxes, file folders or documents, indexes of various types, card catalogs, computerized databases, and standardized summary descriptions. Based on available resources and the nature of its holdings, each repository should strive to develop a unique set of finding aids that will provide the best possible access.

The primary components of a repository's descriptive program are inventories or registers. These documents provide an overview of the collection, together with a description of each record series. The following components are typically included: (1) introductory information, including collection name and number, repository name and address, donor acknowledgments, and special instructions; (2) brief organizational history or individual biography; (3) scope and contents note, a narrative summary description of the records, including particular areas of richness, gaps in documentation, and relationship of the records to other records and subjects, and overall arrangement; (4) series descriptions, including series number and title, dates, quantity, physical format, and information summarizing the activity or function documented by the records, strengths and weaknesses, any restrictions, condition of the records, and information on arrangement; (5) container lists, enumerating folders or other file units in each box, whenever possible utilizing the original folder titles; (6) index to the contents of the inventory, if necessary; and (7) appendices, when appropriate, providing supplementary information (Miller, 1990).

The United States Machine-Readable Cataloging format for archives and manuscripts, USMARC AMC, provides a standard format for the exchange of information on archives and manuscript collections. This standard descriptive tool provides a structure for listing information on groups of records, which can then be shared through national bibliographic utilities such as the Research Libraries Information Network (RLIN) and the Online Computer Library Center (OCLC). Whether or not a new program has computer capabilities, it is important that descriptive practices be developed in such a way that information can be easily converted to USMARC AMC format for future information sharing. While the USMARC AMC format provides a list of information to be included, *Archives, Personal Papers and Manuscripts* (APPM) provides the rules for how information is to be recorded. This cataloging manual provides guidance in describing historical materials "in a manner and style compatible with the description of other library materials." The reference list contains additional resources on standardized descriptive tools.

Preservation

As records are examined and handled during the process of accessioning and arranging, basic preservation measures should be taken. Metal fasteners, paper clips, and rubber bands are damaging to paper documents, and should routinely be removed. Folded documents should be gently unfolded and smoothed flat. Fragile documents should be placed in separate acid-free folders. Careful photocopying of newspaper clippings and other deteriorating documents onto acid-free paper may also be necessary to reduce handling. Some materials, too valuable and fragile to photocopy, should be set aside for additional preservation measures. Acid-free enclosures, including file folders, boxes of various sizes, and specialized enclosures for photographs and other nonpaper records, should replace existing folders and boxes. Each folder must be clearly labeled in pencil, and numbered systematically based on the arrangement plan. Boxes, cabinets, and shelving must also be clearly and systematically labeled and recorded to ensure meticulous tracking of all materials.

The storage environment frequently must be altered to maximize the life of historical and rare materials. In general, minimizing fluctuation in temperature and humidity, and low levels of lighting are desirable. Specific temperature, humidity, and lighting guidelines are available, and should be consulted as part of the program-planning process. Insects, environmental pollutants, and dust are also potentially damaging to records, and provision must be made to reduce damage from these elements as well. Well-designed plans for increasing security from theft, and for coping with environmental disasters such as fire and flooding are essential components of the total program. These subjects are thoroughly covered elsewhere, as indicated in the references at the end of the chapter, and Chapter 8 is devoted solely to preservation issues.

Access

The materials held in a special collections program are by nature rare or one-of-a-kind. Making materials available for research use is the program's primary focus, yet the materials must be protected. Access, then, refers to the "terms and conditions of availability of records or information maintained by an archives for examination and consultation by researchers" (Pederson, 1987, p. 189). Policies and procedures must be developed to protect records and uphold donor agreements and restrictions, while making them available for use. An access policy should be clearly stated and available to potential users of historical materials. This should include a general statement on the nondiscriminatory availability of records for research use, and address confidentiality, protection of privacy, and donor restrictions. It should also include or refer to specific guidelines for the use of the records. Such guidelines typically restrict the use of records to a specific on-site physical location, specify the materials a researcher may bring into the research area, provide for user registration, and address copying and copyright issues (Pederson, 1987). Research agreements may also be developed to formalize the terms agreed upon by the repository and the user. Archives, manuscript collections, and artifacts do not typically circulate to users or to other lending institutions, although provision might be made for the lending of materials for historical exhibits and other specific purposes, depending on the mission of the archives. In these cases, policies and procedures, including careful documentation, should be developed to minimize risk of loss or damage.

Reference Services

Another component of a special collections program is reference services. The researcher often needs to be oriented to the unique nature of special collections materials and instructed in the use of finding aids to identify relevant materials. Box and folder lists may need to be carefully reviewed to determine the relevance of a collection to the research topic, and often the researcher will need to be guided to other repositories for additional information. The definitive print resource for locating repositories is the *National Union Catalog of Manuscript Collections* (NUCMC), published by the Library of Congress since 1959. More recently, records on historical collections have been entered into RLIN and OCLC, the national bibliographic utilities. Because these online databases are not typically available for public use, searches may need to be included as reference services. The World Wide Web is another tool to utilize in the search of repositories with holdings that may contain information on the research topic; the volume of finding aids and repository information available there is growing rapidly, and many repositories provide e-mail response to reference queries. Although the volume of primary source materials available online is very small, using the Internet to locate repositories and obtain information about holdings can save the researcher both time and the expense of travel.

234

CONCLUSION

It is encouraging that there is growing interest and enthusiasm for the history of the profession within the nursing community. Thanks to the efforts of countless nurses, historians, and nursing organizations, there is a growing body of primary source material documenting the profession of nursing. Care must be taken to develop formal programs to ensure these materials are preserved and made available to researchers. This chapter has given a very brief overview of the issues involved in developing a special collections program to maintain archives, manuscript collections, artifacts, and rare books. Developing a program to manage these historical materials can be an exciting adventure.

As with any specialized area, there is a defined body of knowledge to assist in this process. The list of resource references at the end of this chapter is a basic guide to this body of knowledge. Some of the books and articles listed provide a theoretical framework; others offer step-by-step, practical assistance. Publications of the Society of American Archivists (SAA) Archival Fundamentals Series are highly recommended. Furthermore, professional associations offer additional access to both the body of knowledge and the details of practical application; and the small sample of providers of archival supplies are yet another source of assistance. And do not hesitate to tap into the vast experience of professional archivists, records managers, and nursing librarians who have developed programs. Personal contact with a professional who has worked with historical nursing records will provide a wealth of information as well as encouragement and inspiration.

REFERENCES

McCall, N., & Mis, L. A. (Eds.). (1995). *Designing archival programs to advance knowledge in the health fields.* Baltimore: Johns Hopkins University Press.

Miller, F. M. (1990). *Arranging and describing archives and manuscripts.* Chicago: The Society of American Archivists. (SAA Archival Fundamentals Series)

Pederson, A. (Ed.). (1987). *Keeping archives.* Sydney: Australian Society of Archivists Incorporated.

State Archives and Records Administration. (1988). *Strengthening New York's historical records programs: A self study guide.* Albany, NY: Author.

Wilsted, T., & Nolte, W. (1991). *Managing archival and manuscript repositories.* Chicago: The Society of American Archivists. (SAA Archival Fundamentals Series)

Yakel, E. (1994). *Starting an archives.* Metuchen, NJ: Scarecrow Press.

RESOURCE REFERENCES

Bellardo, L., & Bellardo, L. L. (1992). *A glossary for archivists, manuscript curators, and records managers.* Chicago: The Society of American Archivists. (SAA Archival Fundamentals Series)

Betz, E. (1982). *Graphic materials: Rules for describing original items and historical collections.* Washington, DC: Library of Congress.

Depew, J. N. (1991). *A library, media, and archival preservation handbook.* Santa Barbara, CA: ABC-CLIO, Inc.

Ellis, J. (Ed.). (1993). *Keeping archives* (2nd rev. ed.). New Providence, NJ: D. W. Thorpe.

Fortson, J. (1992). *Disaster planning and recovery: A how-to-do-it manual for librarians and archivists.* New York: Neal-Schuman.

Ham, F. G. (1992). *Selecting and appraising archives and manuscripts.* Chicago: The Society of American Archivists. (SAA Archival Fundamental Series)

Hensen, S. L. (1989). *Archives, personal papers, and manuscripts: A cataloging manual for archival repositories, historical societies, and manuscript libraries* (2nd ed.). Chicago: The Society of American Archivists.

Hill, E. (1982). *The preparation of inventories.* (Staff Information Paper 14.) Washington, DC: National Archives and Records Service.

Krizack, J. D. (Ed.). (1994). *Documentation planning for the U.S. health care system.* Baltimore: Johns Hopkins University Press.

Matters, M. (1990). *Introduction to the USMARC format for archival and manuscripts control.* Chicago: The Society of American Archivists.

National Historical Publications and Records Commission. (1988). *Directory of archives and manuscript repositories in the United States* (2nd ed.). Phoenix, AZ: Oryz Press.

Ogden, S. (Ed.). (1992). *Preservation of library & archival materials: A manual.* Andover, MA: Northeast Document Conservation Center.

O'Toole, J. M. (1990). *Understanding archives and manuscripts.* Chicago: The Society of American Archivists. (SAA Archival Fundamentals Series)

Penni, I., Pennix, G., & Coulson, J. (1994). *Records management handbook* (2nd ed.). Brookfield, VT: Ashgate.

Pennsylvania State University. (1996). *Procedures manual: A guide to managing an institutional archive utilizing flow-charts* (rev. ed.). State College, PA: Author.

Pugh, M. J. (1992). *Providing reference services for archives and manuscripts.* Chicago: The Society of American Archivists. (SAA Archival Fundamentals Series)

Ritzenthaler, M. L. (1993). *Preserving archives and manuscripts.* Chicago: The Society of American Archivists. (SAA Archival Fundamentals Series)

Schwartz, C., & Hernon, P. (1993). *Records management and the library: Issues and practices.* Norwood, NJ: ABLEX.

SUGGESTED READINGS

Blodgett, J. (1996). Developing cooperative archives to meet the needs of small institutions. *Resource Sharing & Information Networks, 11*(1/2), 59–68.

McCue, M. P., Poole, C., & Foster E. C. (1989). Establishing hospital archives. *Hospital Topics, 07*(5), 33–36.

Paulson, B. A. (1989). Developing a preservation policy and procedure statement for a health sciences library. *Bulletin of the Medical Library Association, 77,* 293–298.

Weinberg, D. M. (1993). Documenting nursing and health care history in the mid-Atlantic region. *Bulletin of the Medical Library Association, 81,* 29–37.

Yakel, E. (1994). *Starting an archives.* Metuchen, NJ: Scarecrow Press. An excellent overview on the process of initiating an archives program, this manual includes a helpful bibliographical essay, lists of archival organizations, and sample forms.

NATIONAL ORGANIZATIONS

American Association for the History of Nursing (AAHN)
Box 90803
Washington, DC 20090
Publications: *Nursing History Review; Bulletin*

American Association for State and Local History (AASLH)
172 Second Avenue North, Suite 102
Nashville, TN 37201
(615) 255-2971
Publications: *History News; History News Dispatch*

Association of Records Managers
  and Administrators (ARMA)
4200 Somerset Drive, Suite 215
Prairie Village, KA 66208
(913) 341-3808
Publication: *Records Management
  Quarterly*

Society of American Archivists
  (SAA)
600 South Federal, Suite 504
Chicago, IL 60605
(312) 922-0140
Publications: *American Archivist;
  Archival Outlook*

ARCHIVAL SUPPLIES
AND EQUIPMENT

Gaylord Bros.
P.O. Box 4901
Syracuse, NY 13221

Light Impressions
439 Monroe Avenue, P. O. Box 940
Rochester, NY 14603

The Hollinger Corporation, Archival
  Division
P.O. Box 8360
Fredricksburg, VA 22404

University Products
P.O. Box 101
Holyoke, MA 01041

NATIONAL AND REGIONAL
NURSING REPOSITORIES

Center for History of Nursing
Foundation of NYSNA
2113 Western Avenue
Guilderland, NY 12084
(518) 456-7858

Center for Nursing Historical
  Inquiry
University of Virginia Health
  Sciences Center
McLeod Hall
University of Virginia,
  Charlottesville
Charlottesville, VA 22903
(804) 924-0131

Center for the Study of the History
  of Nursing
University of Pennsylvania
School of Nursing, Nursing
  Education Building
Philadelphia, PA 19104
(215) 898-4502

Midwest Nursing History Research
  Center
University of Illinois, Chicago,
  College of Nursing
845 S. Damen Avenue
Chicago, IL 60612
(312) 996-7840

Nursing Archives
Mugar Memorial Library
Boston University
771 Commonwealth Avenue
Boston, MA 02215
(617) 353-3696

Special Collections
Milbank Memorial Library
Teachers College, Columbia
  University
New York, NY 10027
(212) 678-4104

8

Preservation

Karen Sinkule, AMLS

The goal of preserving library and archival materials is to extend their usable life. Preservation is a generic term that encompasses a wide range of activities directed toward current as well as older materials, those intended to last for a limited time, as well as those that are to be retained permanently. While some preservation measures are expensive, many no-cost and low-cost steps can be taken to extend the life of collection materials. The terms *library* and *archive* are used here in a general sense. Library suggests a collection made up largely, but not exclusively, of published materials, while archive suggests one made up largely of unpublished documents and records. Library and archival materials are found in all kinds of information and resource centers, large and small.

At several points in this chapter, the reader is encouraged to seek the advice of a preservation professional. For a fee, consultation services are available from professional consultants in this specialty area. Such services may also be available at no cost at the local, state, or regional level. In addition, readers with preservation questions related to health sciences collections may contact the Preservation and Collection Management Section, National Library of Medicine, 8600 Rockville Pike, Bethesda, MD, 20894; telephone: (301) 496-8124; Fax: (301) 435-2922; e-mail: pres@occshost.nlm.nih.gov.

Karen Sinkule

ENVIRONMENTAL CONSIDERATIONS

Most materials in library and archival collections are subject to chemical deterioration. Over time, acidic paper becomes brittle through oxidation, hydrolysis, and other reactions that break down the links between the cellulose fibers that make up the paper. In photographic materials, chemical deterioration causes fading and physical deformation. Deterioration in organic materials is inevitable, but the rate at which it occurs varies greatly depending on the makeup of the materials and the storage environment: Acidic paper deteriorates much more quickly than alkaline paper; nitrate- and acetate-based photographic formats deteriorate much more quickly than polyester-based formats. Higher temperatures cause molecules to react more rapidly with each other, hastening chemical breakdown, and high humidity promotes hydrolysis reactions and encourages mold growth and insect activity. Light and pollutants also contribute to deterioration.

While institutions can do little to control the makeup of the materials in their collections, they can take steps to improve the storage environment. Maintaining good environmental conditions is, in the long run, more cost-effective than any other preservation measure because it can prevent much of the damage that makes individual treatment of items necessary.

Temperature and Humidity

For the chemical stability of collections, the lower the temperature the better. Lower relative humidity is also better, although extremely low relative humidity, which can occur in buildings with central heating in the winter, can lead to desiccation and embrittlement. Ideal temperature and humidity levels vary depending on the type of material being stored. For example, recommended levels for photographic materials are generally lower than those for paper-based materials.

Fluctuations in relative humidity cause materials to expand and contract. Such dimensional changes accelerate deterioration and can cause paper to cockle, ink to flake, book covers to warp,

242

and photograph emulsions to crack. Therefore, it is important to choose relative humidity levels that can be sustained with relatively small fluctuations. And because temperature affects relative humidity, changes in temperature should be minimized as much as possible.

In setting target temperature and humidity levels, factors other than what is best for the collection must be considered. When people and collections occupy the same space, for example, compromises must be made for human comfort. Patterns of use, the value of the materials, and retention objectives will also influence the choice of environmental boundaries. Local climatic conditions, the constraints of existing buildings and environmental control systems, and cost considerations may dictate what can and cannot be achieved and sustained.

According to the *Environmental Guidelines for the Storage of Paper Records,* a technical report sponsored by the National Information Standards Organization, suggested levels for temperature and relative humidity are as follows.

	Temperature (°F)	Relative Humidity (%)
Combined stack and user areas	70 (maximum)[a]	30–50[b]
Stack areas where people are excluded except for access and retrieval	65 (maximum)[a]	30–50[b]
Optimum preservation stacks	35–65[c]	30–50[b]
Maximum daily fluctuation	+/–2	+/–3
Maximum monthly drift	3	3

[a] These values assume that 70°F is about the minimum comfort temperature for reading, and 65°F the minimum for light physical activity. Each institution can make its own choice.

[b] A *specific value* of relative humidity within this range should be maintained +/–3%, depending on the climatic conditions in the local geographic area or facility limitations.

[c] A *specific temperature* within this range should be maintained +/–2°F. The specific temperature chosen depends on how much an organization is willing to invest in order to achieve a given life expectancy for its records.

Table reprinted with permission from: Wilson, W. K. (1995). *Environmental Guidelines for the Storage of Paper Records.* (NISO-TR01-1995). Bethesda, MD: NISO Press, p. 2.

Maximums of 70 degrees Fahrenheit and 50 percent relative humidity are recommended to minimize the risk of mold growth. Fluctuation ranges of +/−1 degrees Fahrenheit and +/−2 percent relative humidity can be achieved by a well-constructed facility with an excellent HVAC (heating, ventilation, air-conditioning) system and competent technical oversight. A fluctuation range of +/−5 percent relative humidity may be a more reasonable expectation if circumstances are less than ideal. Custom equipment is needed to maintain temperatures below about 65 degrees Fahrenheit.

The benefits of improving temperature and relative humidity conditions are significant. In general, the rate of deterioration can be cut in half with each decrease in temperature of 18 degrees Fahrenheit. The Image Permanence Institute has developed a methodology for estimating the expected usable lifetime of inherently unstable materials such as acidic paper and color slides given various combinations of temperature and relative humidity. According to its research, at 82 degrees Fahrenheit and 75 percent relative humidity, the life expectancy of inherently unstable materials is 9 years; at 72 degrees and 50 percent, 33 years; and at 52 degrees and 30 percent, 243 years (Reilly, Nishimura, & Zinn, 1995).

Ideally, every collection would be stored under stable temperature and humidity conditions appropriate to the nature of the collection and its use. Facilities with less than ideal conditions may be faced with costly improvements, exacerbated by the substantial effort required to convince administrators that improving the storage environment is warranted. Even when administrators are supportive, funding for needed improvements may not be available immediately or even in the forseeable future. Fortunately, in the meantime, many no-cost and low-cost measures can be taken to improve the storage environment. The most valuable materials can be moved to areas with the most desirable conditions. Heating and air-conditioning systems can receive routine maintenance, and filters can be changed regularly. If there is no central air-conditioning, room air conditioners can be used to mitigate extreme heat; portable dehumidifiers can be used in smaller enclosed storage areas. Additional steps can be taken to minimize temperature and humidity fluctuations: Heating and air-conditioning systems should not be turned off over weekends and holidays; windows and doors should be kept closed, and windows should be covered; protective enclosures such as custom-made clamshell boxes can be provided for especially valuable materials.

Light

Cellulose in paper, cloth, and other materials is degraded by photooxidation, a process that weakens the bonds that hold the cellulose fibers together and eventually causes them to break. Photooxidation also causes fading of ink and bindings and bleaching or darkening of paper. Discoloration is especially severe for paper with a high lignin content, such as newsprint. Photooxidation is enhanced by sulfur dioxide and nitrogen dioxide, and accelerates with increases in relative humidity. The chemical processes started by exposing an object to light can continue even after the object is returned to dark storage.

The amount of damage light causes depends on length of exposure, the intensity of the light, and the capacity of the material to absorb radiant energy. Short exposure to high-intensity light is as damaging as long exposure to low-intensity light. Light damage is cumulative, so it is desirable to control the total amount of exposure an object receives. For paper and other light-sensitive materials, light levels should not exceed 55 lux (5-foot candles); for less sensitive materials, they should not exceed 165 lux (15-foot candles). Light from the ultraviolet portion of the spectrum is the most harmful to collections, and the most damaging source of ultraviolet light is sunlight through window glass, more so than direct sunlight alone, and should be avoided if possible. Florescent lamps are the second most damaging source of light, in contrast to incandescent lamps, which have a very small ultraviolet component.

Damage from sunlight can be eliminated by covering windows in collection areas with curtains, shades, or blinds that completely block the sun. Skylights can be covered or painted with titanium dioxide or zinc white pigments that reflect light and absorb UV radiation. UV-filtering plastic films or Plexiglas can reduce (but not eliminate) UV radiation passing through windows and skylights.

Damage from florescent bulbs can be reduced by using UV-filtering light fixtures, special low-UV bulbs, or UV-filtering sleeves over regular bulbs. Filters that exclude wavelengths below about 415 nm are desirable, because they cut out ultraviolet light but do not absorb enough of the visible spectrum to change the color of the object being viewed. Controlling UV exposure is absolutely essential for rare book areas and exhibit cases. Finally, because filtering materials are not effective indefinitely, they need to be tested periodically.

Indirect (reflected) lighting is better than direct lighting because the reflecting surface absorbs some of the ultraviolet light. If possible, storage areas should be kept dark when not in use. Time or motion-detection switches can be installed to turn off lights automatically.

Air Quality

Sulfur dioxide, nitrogen dioxide, and ozone are the principal gaseous contaminants in most archives and libraries. These gases catalyze harmful chemical reactions that lead to the formation of acids, which in turn break down the structure of paper, leather, and other materials. Black soot (primarily from vehicle exhaust fumes) and gray dust (which is usually a combination of soot and particles from ceiling tiles and other objects) are the principal particulate contaminants. They can abrade, soil, and disfigure materials, and carry acids and mold spores into collections.

The removal of gaseous and particulate contaminants requires special equipment not found in most buildings. Gaseous pollutants can be removed by chemical filters, wet scrubbers, or a combination of both. Particulate matter can be removed with a variety of filters depending on the size of the particles to be removed and the level of effectiveness desired. Because heating and air-conditioning systems in general and air-quality equipment in particular vary greatly in complexity and effectiveness, an experienced environmental engineer should be consulted for recommendations specific to the facility and local conditions. Regular system maintenance, including replacement of filters, is essential.

Biological Agents

The biological agents that do the most damage to collections are mold, insects, and rodents. Mold can be a serious problem both for collections and people. Dormant mold spores are present everywhere, all the time. They can be killed only by extremely high heat, which would itself damage collection materials, or by chemicals, which are hazardous to people. Mold growth can be discouraged by controlling temperature and humidity, maintaining good air circulation, keeping storage areas clean, and regularly inspecting air conditioning systems for mold. Ideally, the relative humidity should never rise above 50 percent, because with higher relative humidity, the risk of active mold growth increases. Mold growth is especially likely when a water-related emergency causes materials to get wet.

If a mold outbreak occurs, the affected materials should be isolated immediately. If wet, moldy materials should be air-dried or commercially vacuum freeze-dried. Once dry, any mold residue should be cleaned with a soft brush or a portable vacuum cleaner with a nondamaging brush attachment. Cleaning of mold residue should be done outdoors, away from entrances and air intake vents to prevent mold spores from being reintroduced into storage areas. If a vacuum cleaner is used, it should also be emptied outdoors. Brushes and vacuum cleaner bags should be washed in hot soapy water. Moldy items can be wrapped thoroughly in plastic and frozen in a household-type freezer, which will not kill the mold, but will stabilize the wet materials and prevent further mold growth while plans for recovery are made. Gloves, protective coverings, and a respirator should be worn whenever handling moldy materials. People sensitive to mold should avoid moldy materials because repeated exposure may increase their sensitivity. A preservation expert should be contacted for advice on how to treat a mold outbreak. Rare or fragile materials that have become moldy should be referred to a conservator for cleaning.

Pests such as insects and rodents are attracted by food remains and clutter. If they find their way into libraries and archives, they may stay to feed on materials in the collection. To discourage pests, keep storage areas clean and free of clutter. Prohibit food, beverages, and houseplants in collection areas. Empty garbage cans daily. Keep windows and doors closed as much as possible. Keep plantings at least 18 inches away from the building. If possible, check all materials entering the building for evidence of infestation, including materials being added to the collection, materials returned after circulation, and supplies and packing materials. Routine inspections by a pest control specialist are recommended.

If an infestation occurs, isolate the affected items and adjacent materials. For reasons of staff safety, it is advisable to hire a pest control specialist to catch rodents or apply insecticides. If chemicals are to be used, ensure they do not come in contact with collection materials. Materials infested with insects can be treated by freezing them to approximately minus 30 degrees Fahrenheit. As an extra precaution, infested materials can be frozen, allowed to thaw to room temperature, then frozen to minus 30 degrees a second time.

Environmental Monitoring

A variety of equipment is available for measuring temperature, relative humidity, and light levels. Equipment for measuring humidity includes reversible humidity strips, nonreversible high/low strips, hygrometers, and wet-bulb/dry-bulb sling and aspirating psychrometers. For ease of use and reasonable cost, the two best choices are reversible humidity strips (under $2), which are very accurate particularly when used to measure very high and low humidities, and battery-operated aspirating psychrometers (under $200). Temperature can be measured with a variety of thermometers (bimetal strip, alcohol, or mercury), thermocouples, and thermistors, all of which are relatively inexpensive and accurate to +/−1 degree Fahrenheit. Recording hygrothermographs produce a paper graph of both temperature and humidity levels over time. The most desirable hygrothermographs have a humidity scale that is at least one-half of the chart; multiple speeds with at least one-day, seven-day, and 30-day rotations; easy one-step/one-tool recalibration; cartridge-type pens; and the longest possible hygrometer hairs. Recording hygrothermographs are more expensive (about $700) than other measuring equipment, but they are highly recommended because they are relatively simple to operate, can be read directly to check recent conditions and thereby identify problems that require immediate attention, and provide a record of fluctuations over time. Computerized temperature and humidity sensors, or data loggers, are also available ($600–$1,000). These have more sophisticated capabilities for processing and displaying data than a hygrothermograph, but require a computer, some computer expertise, and unless they have a real-time readout of recent conditions, are not as convenient for identifying current problems.

To begin a temperature and humidity monitoring program, identify all of the specific locations at which recordings will be taken. Include locations that are known to have extreme conditions, that are controlled by different air-handling systems, that house especially valuable materials, and that are used for exhibits. At the outset, take readings in each location at several different times of day, including evenings and weekends if possible. Once patterns of fluctuations are apparent, plan a manageable schedule of readings to establish baseline data for a year, concentrating on problem locations but also including some regular readings in each major collection storage area to identify seasonal trends. If hygrothermographs are used, check them daily to see if there have been any major fluctuations indicating a problem that requires immediate attention. Periodically check the accuracy of equipment by taking simultaneous readings using two different devices.

Light levels can be checked with a lux/foot candlelight meter, which is accurate at low light levels (about $120), or a single-lens reflex camera with a built-in light meter. Ultraviolet light can be measured with a UV monitor (over $1,000). A less accurate but much less expensive tool for measuring ultraviolet light is a textile fading strip (about $20 for 6). Collection materials exposed to outside light should be measured at different times of day and at different seasons. Light in collection areas with florescent bulbs should be measured every six months to determine if the UV filters or sleeves remain effective.

The presence of particulate contaminants can be checked with white gloves ($5). Gaseous contaminants can be evaluated using electronic detectors or corrosion coupons (about $500), which turn or corrode to different colors depending on the type of contaminant present.

In addition to monitoring environmental conditions, buildings should be inspected regularly to identify potentially damaging conditions and to check for evidence of mold or pest infestation. If water leaks are known or suspected to be a problem, water sensors can be installed. Sensors that set off an alarm at a central monitoring station are effective but quite expensive to install. A less reliable but much less expensive measure is to use local water alarms ($20 each). Sticky traps can be set to identify areas of insect activity.

By monitoring environmental conditions on an ongoing basis, you can identify problems promptly so that timely corrective action can be taken; establish baseline conditions; and document daily, weekly, and seasonal fluctuations. These data will be useful when dealing with building maintenance staff and repairpersons or when making a case for installing better air systems. Armed with documentation of the extent of your facility's problems, you can work to educate administrators, building engineers, and maintenance staff that libraries and archives have special environmental requirements and that maintenance of proper conditions is the single most important element in preserving collections.

STORAGE AND HANDLING

Good storage and handling practices reduce physical damage to collection materials. While many recommended practices are common-sense measures that can be implemented at low cost, they are all too often overlooked. Some of the recommended storage supplies can be expensive, but most items are available from several different vendors so it is worthwhile to compare prices.

When selecting supplies, it is important to read product descriptions carefully. Terms such as *archival* and *preservation* have little meaning on their own, and it is necessary to check the composition of storage supplies to ensure they are suitable. To preservation specialists, *archival-quality* means a set of properties that vary for different types of materials, but that have in common the effect of reducing the damaging impact of poor environment or handling. Archival-quality paper is often referred to as "permanent."[1] For storage of most types of material, paper enclosures should have a low lignin content[2] and be alkaline-buffered.[3] A few types of material, such as blueprints and color photographs and negatives, may be damaged by alkaline chemicals. For these materials, it is safest to use unbuffered, acid-neutral, low-lignin enclosures. A reasonably accurate test of paper acidity can be made with inexpensive pH testing pens, which are used to make a small mark on the paper to be tested. The mark will turn different colors depending on the level of acidity or alkalinity. When in doubt about the kind of storage enclosures to purchase, consult a preservation specialist.

Storing Books

Shelving should be spaced so that books can stand upright with spines facing out. If this is not possible, books should be shelved with the spine resting horizontally on the shelf. Books should not be shelved on their fore-edge, because this encourages the textblock to separate from its cover. Books should not extend past the edge of the shelf. This helps to prevent items from being

---

[1] In *Permanence of Paper for Publications and Documents in Libraries and Archives*, the National Information Standards Organization (1992) requires that to be considered "permanent," uncoated paper must have a pH in the range of 7.5 to 10 (pH 7.0 to 10 for the core of coated papers), have a minimum alkaline reserve equivalent to 2 percent calcium carbonate, have no more than 1 percent lignin content, and meet certain tear-resistance requirements.

[2] Lignin is a natural component of woody materials that darkens when exposed to light. Low-lignin paper (often referred to as "lignin-free" in product descriptions) may be made from substances that contain little lignin, such as cotton and linen, or from substances that have had the lignin removed.

[3] Buffering is a process by which an alkaline substance, usually calcium carbonate, is added to raise the pH of paper in order to counteract the detrimental effects of acids that may be present in the material being stored and pollutants in the environment. For storage enclosures, an alkaline "reserve" equivalent to 2 to 3 percent calcium carbonate by weight and resulting in a pH of 8.5 or higher is recommended.

knocked off the shelf, as well as reducing fading of spines and covers and the risk of damage from overhead water leaks. Books should be held upright with bookends, but they should not be packed so tightly that they cannot be removed easily or so loosely that they lean.

Bookends should be large enough to support at least half the height of most books and should have a smooth, nondamaging surface. The vertical part of the bookend should have a broad edge to prevent it from knifing into textblocks and thus damaging pages. Wire bookends that hang from the top of the shelf are not recommended.

Oversized books often have bindings that are weak in proportion to their size and weight, and require special shelving. They should be stored flat on shelves that are wide enough to support them fully. No more than three or four volumes should be stacked on top of each other.

Book trucks should be easy to maneuver and be loaded so that weight is evenly distributed. Books should be placed upright with spines out and be supported by bookends, or placed flat in low stacks.

Storing Flat Paper

Documents and manuscripts in good condition should be unfolded and stored flat. If items are brittle or fragile and cannot be unfolded without damage, reformat them or consult a conservator for advice on treatment before storing. All damaging fasteners, such as staples, paper clips, pins, rubber bands, and string, should be removed unless they are so firmly embedded in the paper that attempting to remove them is likely to cause damage. If absolutely necessary, clips and staples can be replaced with nonrusting ones. If paper clips are used, a small piece of acid-free paper should be folded in half over the top of the document and under the clip to prevent creasing. Acidic envelopes, folders, or other enclosures should be replaced unless they have intrinsic value. Removable "sticky" notes and tabs should be removed.

Flat paper should be stored in alkaline-buffered, low-lignin file folders or in alkaline-buffered, low-lignin envelopes with inner sleeves, which help to prevent damage as sheets are inserted and removed. Ideally, no more than 10 to 15 sheets should be stored in a folder or envelope. If possible, materials of different sizes and weights should not be stored together. Pencil should be used for handwritten labels since many inks are water-soluble and can fade.

Documents on highly acidic paper, such as newsprint, should not be in direct contact with other documents because acid will migrate to adjacent nonacidic materials and cause them to become discolored and brittle. Acidic materials should be interleaved with alkaline paper and stored separately or be placed in polyester sleeves. If highly acidic materials are to be retained for any length of time, they should be photocopied onto permanent paper or microfilmed.

Damaged, fragile, and brittle documents may be placed in clear polyester sleeves, sealed on two adjacent edges. Such sleeves will allow most items to be handled and read without further damage. However, because polyester film creates static electricity, it cannot be used for items that may powder or flake, such as chalk and charcoal drawings, blueprints, and photographs with damaged surfaces.

Folders and envelopes should be kept in alkaline, low-lignin document storage boxes of similar size. Whenever possible, all folders in a box should be the same size and should fill the box comfortably without being overfull. Alkaline boards can be used to fill boxes that are not quite full. Boxes may be stored upright if the materials inside are well supported and will not slump in the box. Boxes may be stored flat if their contents are not well supported, providing that very heavy items are not resting on top of smaller or more fragile items in the box. Boxes should not be stacked more than two high. As an alternative to boxes, folders and envelopes may be kept in cabinets designed for hanging file folders. The hanging file folders should be alkaline and should not be overfilled.

Large flat sheets, such as maps and architectural drawings, are best stored flat in the drawers of a map case or in large alkaline, low-lignin boxes. Items should be placed in acid-free folders sized to fit the drawer or box, because folders that are smaller than their container tend to shift, jam, or allow their contents to slide out. No more than a few items should be stored in one folder. Fragile or acidic materials should be interleaved with alkaline paper. (Blueprints, however, must be stored in unbuffered, pH-neutral folders because alkaline buffers can cause them to fade or discolor.) If flat storage is not possible, oversized material in good condition can be rolled. Items may be stored inside a tube, and wrapped in alkaline paper or polyester film if the tube is acidic. They may also be placed in a polyester sleeve, rolled around the outside of a tube, and tied loosely with linen, cotton, or polyester flat tape. Choose tubes with a wide diameter and several inches longer than the material inside.

Storing Photographs

If possible, each photograph should each be stored in its own enclosure to decrease the possibility of processing chemicals migrating from image to image and to reduce handling. Prints and negatives should not be stored in the same enclosure because of the possibility of transfer of harmful chemicals from one to the other. Enclosures should be made of nondamaging plastic or paper. Glassine, a traditional material for storing negatives and interleaving, is no longer recommended because it loses its translucency and absorbs acids and moisture.

A plastic enclosure allows the photograph to be seen without being removed and protects it from moisture and pollutants. However, plastic enclosures have some limitations; in particular, they should not be used if the storage area has high humidity, because they can trap moisture inside and cause sticking. Neither should they be used for negatives on cellulose nitrate or acetate film, because they can accelerate deterioration. Finally, the possibility of static electricity makes plastic enclosures unsuitable for photos that have flaking or lifting emulsions, and they may be difficult to write on and to support in a storage box. Despite these disadvantages, plastic enclosures are preferred over paper envelopes for photographs that are intended for use, because they protect photos from dirty hands and other damage that might occur while being handled. Types of plastic acceptable for long-term storage include polyester, uncoated polypropylene, and high-density polyethylene. Polyvinyl chloride (PVC) and cellulose triacetate are not acceptable.

Paper enclosures protect photographic materials from light, prevent accumulation of moisture and harmful gases, do not cause sticking, and are easy to write on. However, because the image cannot be seen without being removed, paper enclosures increase the risk of abrasion, damage from dirty hands, and misfiling. All paper enclosures should be made of nonacidic, low-lignin paper.[4] Buffered paper is recommended for black-and-white photographs and negatives, all nitrate and acetate film, brittle prints, and prints on acidic mounts. Unbuffered paper is recommended for color photographs and negatives, cyanotypes, such as architectural blueprints, dye transfer prints, and albumen prints.

Notations on photographs should be kept to a minimum and written in soft pencil on the back. Negatives should never be marked. Notes should be made on the enclosure before placing the photograph or negative inside. Stainless steel paper clips may be used to attach sleeved photos to accompanying text if care is taken to ensure that the photograph is positioned in the sleeve in such a way that the clip does not apply pressure to it.

Storage Furniture

Dry powder-coated metal shelving and storage cabinets are currently recommended for library and archival materials. Dry powder coatings are electrostatically applied and then baked; they are inert, odorless, and employ no unstable components that can volatilize and interact harmfully with collection materials. Until

---

[4] ANSI IT9.2-1991, *Imaging Media—Photographic Processed Films, Plates, and Papers—Filing Enclosures and Storage Containers* (American National Standards Institute, 1991), describes the characteristics of paper and plastic enclosures that are appropriate for use with photographic materials.

recently, it was recommended that storage furniture have a baked enamel finish, but baked enamel has been found to give off formaldehyde and other harmful volatiles if it is not baked long enough at a high enough temperature. Such off-gassing can be a serious problem if it occurs in an enclosed space, such as a file cabinet or an area with poor air circulation. When purchasing baked enamel storage units, be sure the manufacturer documents that they comply with the American Society of Testing Materials (ASTM) test E-595.

Shelving and storage units made of wood are not recommended because they can emit acids and other harmful substances. Oak is particularly damaging and should be avoided. If wooden furniture must be used, it should be sealed with moisture-borne polyurethane or paint and then be lined with an effective barrier material. Consult a preservation professional for current advice before deciding to treat wood furniture.

Shelving and other storage units should keep collection materials four to six inches off the floor to protect them from dust, feet, and water damage. To improve air circulation and decrease the risk of water damage, do not store collection materials against walls, especially outside walls. Shelving should be strong, smooth, and free of exposed nuts and bolts. It should be adjustable to accommodate books of different sizes. Stack ranges should be bolted to the floor and adequately cross-braced to prevent toppling. Extra care should be taken in shelving books on movable compact shelving to ensure that books are well supported and do not protrude over the end of the shelf in order to prevent them from falling when ranges are moved.

Retrieval and Reshelving

A book should be removed from the shelf by grasping it gently on both sides at midspine with thumb and fingers. If necessary, the books on either side of the desired volume should be pushed back slightly to allow the book to be grasped securely. Books should not be pulled off the shelf by grasping the headcap (top edge of the spine), a common practice that is the cause of most spine damage. When a book is reshelved, the bookend should be moved to make space for the item and then be readjusted. When handling oversized volumes or flat sheets, it is important that they be well supported. Special care is needed when unfolding or unrolling documents. If they resist gentle pressure, they should be referred to a conservator to be humidified and flattened or repaired.

Photographic materials are delicate and easily scratched, torn, creased, or broken. Clean lintless white gloves should be worn whenever handling prints or negatives because oils and chemicals from hands can cause permanent damage. Photographic materials should always be handled by their edges and supported underneath to prevent bending, which can crack the emulsion.

Photocopying

A great deal of damage is done to bound volumes by photocopying. On a standard office copier, volumes must be opened 180 degrees and pressure must be applied to the spine in order to press the text flat against the glass. In volumes with stiff bindings or narrow inner margins, the pressure needed is considerable, thus photocopying often results in broken sewing, cracked adhesive, and detached pages, especially if the paper is brittle. When more than a few pages become detached in one place, they cannot be reattached and the volume must be rebound. If the volume has insufficient inner margins or brittle pages, rebinding may be impossible.

To minimize damage, use photocopiers designed for bound volumes. Such copiers have a glass surface that extends to the edge of the machine, thus permitting volumes to be copied without being opened 180 degrees. They also provide better support for volumes while being copied. Regardless of the type of copier used, bound volumes should be copied one page at a time, without applying pressure to the spine and back of the volume. Some loss of legibility should be tolerated to prevent permanent damage to the volume. Patrons should not be permitted to photocopy rare, fragile, or brittle materials. Staff may copy such material if they judge it to be safe.

Karen Sinkule

Other

Food and drink should be prohibited where collection materials are used. If books are sent out on interlibrary loan, they should be packed in sturdy boxes or strong envelopes with sufficient packing material to ensure that they are well-padded and will not shift during transit. If possible, book drops should be eliminated because they damage materials and can be a fire and vandalism hazard if built into an exterior wall. If they cannot be eliminated, choose the kind with a spring mechanism, make them available only when the facility is closed, and avoid locating them inside the building. Tile floors are recommended for collection storage areas, especially those housing rare or special collections, because tile is easier to keep clean than carpeting.

HOUSEKEEPING

Good housekeeping practices reduce the risk of mold outbreaks, pest infestations, and disfiguration and damage to collections, but it is important that cleaning be carried out with preservation in mind. Routine cleaning of floors and furniture can be done by regular housekeeping staff, providing they work carefully around collection materials and do not use unacceptable cleaning products. Establishing good communication with housekeeping staff is important, and ongoing monitoring is needed to ensure that agreed-upon procedures are followed.

Every library and archive should have a program for cleaning its entire collection every three to eight years. It is important that the cleaning of collection materials be performed by trained staff or contractors, not untrained maintenance personnel, because of the danger of damaging materials, especially if they are rare or fragile. One of the challenges in supervising a stack-cleaning project is motivating staff and convincing them of the importance of their work.

Most cleaning products leave an oily residue and should not be used on any surface where books or other materials are stored or used, because the oil will be transferred to the materials. Whenever water or wax are used in collection areas, care must be taken that they are not splashed onto books.

Tile floors in collection storage areas should be dusted regularly and damp-mopped and waxed as needed. Areas with carpeting should be vacuumed regularly. Shelves and storage cabinets can be vacuumed or dusted with special cloths that attract dirt electrostatically. Such cloths can be washed and reused many times. Other kinds of treated cloths should not be used because of the risk that they will leave a residue. Shelves and storage cabinets can be wiped with a damp cloth if care is taken that surfaces are dry before reshelving materials.

Books can be cleaned carefully with a portable vacuum cleaner that has a filter that traps dust effectively; it should not, however, have such powerful suction that it causes damage to pages or labels. The brush attachment should be soft and nondamaging and covered with cheesecloth to further protect books from abrasion. The cheesecloth should be replaced as soon as it is dirty. Books must be held tightly closed while the edges of the textblock and covers are vacuumed to prevent dirt from being transferred to pages. The insides of books should not be vacuumed. Rare, fragile, or brittle books should be referred to a conservator for cleaning.

Storage boxes can be vacuumed or dusted with an electrostatic cloth. Paper documents in good condition can be lightly dusted with a soft brush. Photographs should be cleaned only by a conservator. Trash cans that may contain food remains should be emptied daily.

BINDING AND OTHER ENCLOSURES

Binding is perhaps the most common preservation activity in libraries and archives. Binding can greatly extend the usable life of materials if wise decisions are made and if newly bound volumes are inspected regularly to ensure the quality of the binder's work. It is worthwhile to visit your binder, or any large binder, to see the operation firsthand. The *Guide to the Library Binding Institute Standard for Library Binding* (Merrill-Oldham & Parisi, 1990) is an excellent source of information about binding vocabulary, methods, and standards. Three main types of binding are available commercially: sewing through the fold, double-fan adhesive, and oversewing. Each of these methods attaches pages together in a different way, and each has advantages and limitations.

Sewing through the fold is always the preferred method of binding, because it is strong, does not cause any loss of inner margins, and allows volumes to open easily and lie flat once opened. Because of its superior openability, volumes sewn through the fold are less likely to be damaged in photocopying than volumes bound using other methods. The limitation of the sewing through the fold method is that it can be used only for materials whose pages are in signatures. (A signature is a group of sheets folded to page size in the center prior to binding.)

Double-fan adhesive binding is one method of binding materials whose pages are individual sheets rather than folded signatures. Its main advantages are that it allows volumes to open easily and lie flat, causes minimal loss of inner margins, and can be used for some brittle paper. Its limitations are that it cannot be used for thick, heavy, or glossy paper or for thick volumes. For double-fan adhesive binding to be durable, it is essential that the proper adhesive is used and applied correctly.

The second method of binding materials whose pages are not in signatures is oversewing. Oversewing is extremely strong and therefore is good for thick or glossy paper, thick volumes, and heavily used materials. Oversewing was once the most common method of library binding, but it has several important disadvantages. Oversewing removes more of the inner margin than other methods, therefore oversewn volumes do not open easily or lie flat when opened. For these reasons, oversewn volumes are difficult to photocopy and are likely to be damaged during copying because of the amount of pressure needed to flatten the volume on the glass. In oversewing, thread pierces each page many times resulting in very strong sewing. While this strength is in some ways an advantage, as the paper becomes brittle, pages are more likely to become detached, and because of the reduced inner margin, many oversewn volumes cannot be rebound.

In addition to these basic binding methods, most commercial binders offer a variety of special services, such as recasing (replacing

covers while keeping the original method of page attachment), rebinding (removing and replacing the sewing or adhesive as well as
the cover), making pockets and boxes, collating and preparing materials, and repairing damage. Every institution that has materials
bound should have a binding contract that specifies how the
choice of binding method is to be made and what specific services
are to be performed, as well as the criteria by which work will be
evaluated. A sample of each binding shipment should be inspected
to ensure the quality of materials and workmanship and the appropriateness of the binding methods chosen.

REPAIR AND CONSERVATION

Each institution needs to decide what its overall approach to repair
and conservation will be, what specific treatments will be performed, and who will perform them. An institution's overall approach may range from no treatment at all to treating individual
items when damage is noted to systematically carrying out a program to assess the overall needs of the collection, set priorities,
and actively identify items to receive treatment. Treatments may
range from simple repairs to complex conservation treatments. Existing staff may be trained to perform treatments, individuals may
be hired on contract to perform treatments on-site, or materials
may be sent to outside vendors.

The decisions an institution makes about the kinds of repair or
conservation to undertake will depend on many factors, including
the nature, use, rarity, value, and intended permanence of materials in the collection, as well as the amount of funding, staffing,
and space available. In many institutions, the approach for general
collection materials focuses on preserving the intellectual content
of a work rather than on retaining it in its original form and on
treating batches of materials that have similar problems. The approach for rare or special collection materials usually focuses on
preservation of the original and treatment of individual items.

Simple repairs that can be performed with a relatively small
amount of training, inexpensive supplies, and minimal space and
equipment include mending paper tears, tipping in detached or

261

replacement pages, tightening and repairing hinges, mending simple cover and spine tears, making wraparound enclosures, tying fragile volumes, encapsulating documents, making book jackets, and binding pamphlets. For general collection materials, such repairs are usually performed in-house.

Intermediate treatments that require more training and more specialized supplies or equipment include removing difficult fasteners, flattening documents in poor condition, making simple custom-fit boxes, recasing books, and performing more complex cover and spine repairs. These types of repairs may be performed in-house by trained staff or contractors or off-site by a commercial vendor.

Complex treatments that require a skilled conservator and specialized supplies and equipment include cleaning paper, deacidifying pages, repairing signatures and sewing structures, performing complicated page repairs, and constructing clamshell boxes and other special enclosures. Such treatments may be done on-site or by a commercial conservation center.

DISASTER PREPAREDNESS

Every library and archive should be prepared for disasters. While relatively few institutions suffer catastrophes, most will experience some kind of emergency that threatens their collection. A disaster preparedness program includes taking steps to prevent disasters, developing a plan for responding to disasters, training staff to assist with disaster recovery, and purchasing disaster recovery supplies and equipment. Many good publications on disaster planning are available. One of the best is *Disaster Planning for Libraries: A How-to-Do-It Manual for Librarians and Archivists* (Fortson, 1992) which includes sample plans, sources of disaster recovery services, and an extensive bibliography.

The greatest hazard faced by libraries and archives is fire. Every institution should have fire-detection and fire-suppression systems. Heat and smoke detectors should be connected to the local fire department or other monitoring station that is staffed 24 hours a day. Automatic water sprinklers currently are considered the best type of fire-suppression system for libraries and archives. Various kinds of sprinklers and detectors are available, and a fire safety engineer familiar with the special needs of libraries and archives can provide advice about the most appropriate type of equipment for your facility. Establishing good communications with local fire officials is beneficial. Fire officials can inspect the condition of fire detection and sprinkler systems, review evacuation plans, and determine whether there are fire hazards that need to be corrected. They can be made aware of the value of the library collection and the importance of extinguishing a fire in the facility with the least amount of water consistent with safety in order to avoid unnecessary water damage to the collection.

The second greatest collection hazard is water. Water damage may occur as a consequence of a fire or flood, but more often is the result of leaks. To minimize the risk of water damage, the building should be inspected regularly, especially the roof, exterior walls, plumbing, and sprinkler systems. Follow-up may be needed to ensure that repairs are made. It is a good idea to check for leaks whenever there are heavy rains, especially in collection areas with a history of leaks; and special attention should be paid when there are construction projects in or near the building. Disasters have a tendency to occur on weekends and holidays, so if possible, the facility should be checked periodically when it is closed. Because disasters cannot always be prevented, institutions should carry insurance against collection damage and loss unless they are self-insured.

Every institution should have a sufficient quantity of recovery supplies and equipment on hand to take care of typical emergencies. Among the most useful supplies are plastic sheeting to protect dry materials, a ladder, a wet vacuum to clean up water, and cartons to pack materials in for transport to freezers or freeze-dry facilities. Corrugated plastic cartons that can be stored flat are particularly good because they will not collapse with the weight of wet material, can be reused, and will not attract insects while being stored. Disaster supplies should be easily accessible; but because they tend to disappear, they need to be checked and replenished regularly.

Having a written disaster plan is invaluable. There are many good models to follow, but every institution needs to develop its own plan based on its collection, physical facilities, and staffing levels. The first step in developing a disaster plan is to identify members of the response team. It is desirable to include individuals who have a knowledge of collection usage and collection strengths as well as building maintenance staff. Responsibility for key aspects of recovery, such as supervising recovery operations, making salvage decisions, and arranging for purchase of services or additional supplies should be assigned in advance. In general, a disaster plan should include the following:

Instructions on what to do immediately when a disaster is discovered.

A telephone tree of people and units to be notified.

Floor plans.

A list of supplies and equipment on hand.

A list of available resources, such as nearby freezer space, sources for additional supplies and equipment, and consultants.

Collection salvage priorities.

Procedures for handling and packing wet materials.

Once the plan is written, it should be distributed to all individuals involved, who should be instructed to keep copies at home as well as at work; staff training should be provided. The plan should be updated at least annually.

There are several key points to remember in responding to a disaster:

1. Establish that the area is safe to enter.
2. Identify the source of the problem and contact appropriate people to correct it.
3. Protect dry materials by moving them or covering them with plastic sheeting.

4. Lower the temperature and humidity, and increase air circulation to reduce the risk of mold growth.

If you are unfamiliar with recovering wet materials, contact a preservation specialist for advice as soon as possible. Wet materials should be taken to a clean, dry area. Most paper-based items can be air-dried if there are not too many of them. Alternatively, most paper-based items can be frozen safely to stabilize them. Frozen materials can subsequently be removed in manageable quantities and air-dried or be shipped frozen for vacuum freeze-drying. Most wet paper-based materials can be recovered successfully, but certain materials, including coated (glossy) paper, flat paper materials that have become really wet, oversized documents, and non-paper formats require special treatment. Obtain expert advice if such materials need to be recovered.

REFORMATTING

Reformatting preserves the intellectual content of an item, rather than the item itself. Libraries and archives may reformat materials to preserve them, improve access to them, or both. The two main methods of reformatting paper-based materials for preservation purposes are microfilming and photocopying. Photographic materials can be reformatted by having them rephotographed or, for some types of negatives, duplicated. Because reformatting photographic materials is expensive and often involves complex decisions, it is essential to obtain expert advice before deciding to do so. Digital imaging is a rapidly developing reformatting technology with great potential for improving access, but at the current time it has limited value as a means of preservation.

Microfilming

Of all the methods of reformatting paper-based materials, microfilming offers the greatest and most assured longevity. If properly processed and stored, microfilm has a life expectancy in excess of 500 years. Microfilming is a stable technology; there are national standards for the composition, production, and storage of microfilm and accepted guidelines for the preparation of materials prior to filming. Microfilm is relatively simple format, requiring only a light source and magnification to be read. It allows deteriorating material to be reformatted once and copies to be made available to multiple users anywhere at any time. Microfilm can be duplicated onto paper and scanned for electronic distribution.

Microfilming has some limitations. High-contrast black-and-white microfilm, the type most commonly used, does not adequately capture information in color or gray tones. Continuous-tone and color microfilms are available that can reproduce gray tones and color with good fidelity, but these types of microfilm are considerably more expensive than high-contrast film, and their use for materials containing both text and color or gray tones can present logistical problems. Because materials being filmed are subjected to a considerable amount of handling, and because the filming process exerts some pressure on bound volumes, filming is likely to cause damage to brittle or fragile materials. The risk of damage is a particular problem for rare or artifactually valuable items, which are to be retained in their original form after filming, thus it is essential to make special arrangements for the filming of such materials. In some cases, such items cannot be filmed because damage would be inevitable.

The microfilming process begins with preparation, which includes making sure that materials are complete and in order, obtaining replacements for missing or illegible material if possible, and producing "targets" to provide bibliographic and other information useful to patrons. Most institutions contract with a vendor for microfilming. It is essential to choose a vendor with experience in producing preservation microfilm from library and archival materials. To ensure that the microfilm produced is of preservation quality, institutions have a responsibility to inspect samples of the microfilm they produce and store the master reels off-site under proper conditions. Entering data about newly produced microfilm in a national bibliographic utility will inform other libraries of its availability and prevent duplicative preservation effort. Institutions considering microfilming for nursing or other biomedical materials should first contact the National Library of Medicine for assistance in determining whether the material has already been filmed or is scheduled for filming by NLM or another library.

Photocopying

The usable life of paper materials in poor condition or on acidic paper can be extended by photocopying them onto alkaline, low-lignin, permanent paper. Double-sided photocopies with wide inner margins are often made so that the photocopies can be bound and shelved in the collection. If desired, color illustrations can be photocopied in color, although the permanence of color photocopies is not assured. Preservation photocopying can be done in-house by trained staff or be contracted out to a vendor. To reduce the risk of damage to the original, copies should be produced using a photocopier designed for copying bound volumes (with glass to the edge) or a digital scanner with a book cradle that allows volumes to be scanned in a face-up position. Photocopying has the advantage of producing a paper product very similar to the original. It is easier to make preservation photocopies or arrange for a vendor to produce them for you than it is to arrange for microfilming. However, unlike microfilm, a photocopied item cannot serve as a "master" that can be stored safely off-site and be used to make an unlimited number of use copies.

Digital Imaging

Digital imaging, or scanning, is a means of capturing and storing images using computer technology. Most types of library and archival material can be scanned, including printed and handwritten text, illustrations, photographic negatives and prints, and microfilm. Digital imaging offers many advantages to users but it has many limitations as a preservation tool.

Because digital images can be manipulated, it is possible to improve the legibility of deteriorated text, insert missing material, or correct other problems that are identified after the initial scanning is completed. Digital data can be indexed to provide a variety of ways of locating individual images: It can be reproduced on optical digital disk, CD-ROM, microfilm, or paper, and thus meet a variety of user preferences and equipment constraints. For libraries and archives, the greatest potential of digital imaging is its ability to provide access to remote information. Scanned images can be mounted on local or national computer networks and distributed to any computer that has access to the network.

While digital imaging is very attractive from a use perspective, it is not so attractive from a preservation perspective. Digital images inevitably will be manipulated, whether to enhance them, compress them for storage or transmission, convert them to a different computer file format, or for other reasons. As a result, scanned images are inherently "unstable" as compared with microform images, which by their nature are unalterable. The mutability of digital data makes it difficult to determine which version of a scanned image is the "master" and therefore the version that needs to be retained and preserved. Because computer hardware and access software are evolving very rapidly, digital images produced and stored using today's equipment and software will become inaccessible unless the data is continually migrated to newer systems. Widely accepted best practices for the capture and archiving of digital images do not exist and are not likely to be developed for some time.

Today, scanning can serve as a preservation tool in certain ways, such as to reduce the handling of original materials and permit them to be stored remotely under better environmental conditions, or to produce paper copies of brittle or fragile materials with less damage than would be caused by photocopying. Scanning can also serve as an adjunct to preservation by providing wider access to materials. But at this time, materials that have been scanned cannot be considered to have been preserved.

SELECTION FOR PRESERVATION

In selecting items for preservation treatment, many factors need to be considered, such as rarity, artifactual or monetary value, condition, importance to the collection or mission of the institution, current use, and potential for future use. Bear in mind that preservation "treatment" is not limited to expensive measures such as conservation or microfilming. Treatment can mean moving the item to an area with better environmental conditions, putting it in an acid-free envelope, or moving it off the floor to protect it from water damage. Even the decision *not* to discard an item is a preservation decision in the sense that the item will still be available for future consideration.

Organizations should give priority to preserving their own publications and records. Archival documents, manuscripts, photographs, pamphlets, posters, and ephemeral materials should receive special consideration for preservation treatment because of their potential uniqueness and research value. Local, regional, and state publications that are not widely held, or if held may not be retained permanently by other institutions, should also be considered for preservation. The National Library of Medicine can provide advice on selecting materials for preservation and on making retention decisions.

CONCLUSION

An institution invests substantial money and time in acquiring materials to meet its information needs. The rate at which these materials deteriorate depends in large part on the ways in which they are stored, handled, and cared for. By following good preservation practices whenever possible, an institution can help to ensure that the materials it has collected remain in usable condition for as long as they are needed.

REFERENCES

American National Standards Institute. (1991). *Imaging media—Photographic processed films, plates, and papers—Filing enclosures and storage containers.* (ANSI IT9.2-1991). New York: American National Standards Institute.

Fortson, J. (1992). *Disaster planning and recovery: A how-to-do-it manual for librarians and archivists.* New York: Neal-Schuman.

Karen Sinkule

Merrill-Oldham, J., & Parisi, P. (1990). *Guide to the library binding institute standard for library binding.* Chicago: American Library Association.

National Information Standards Organization. (1992). *Permanence of paper for publications and documents in libraries and archives.* (ANSI/NISO Z39.48-1992). Bethesda, MD: NISO Press.

Reilly, J. M., Nishimura, D. W., & Zinn, E. (1995). *New tools for preservation: Assessing long-term environmental effects on library and archives collections.* Washington, DC: Commission on Preservation and Access.

Wilson, W. K. (1995). *Environmental guidelines for the storage of paper records.* (NISO-TR01-1995). Bethesda, MD: NISO Press.

RESOURCE REFERENCES

Basic conservation of archival materials: A guide. (1990). Ottawa, Canada: Canadian Council of Archives.

Fortson, J. (1992). *Disaster planning and recovery: A how-to-do-it manual for librarians and archivists.* New York: Neal-Schuman.

Fox, L. L. (Ed.). (1996). *Preservation microfilming: A guide for librarians and archivists* (2nd ed.). Chicago: American Library Association.

Harmon, J. D. (1993). *Integrated pest management in museum, library, and archival facilities.* Indianapolis, IN: Harmon Preservation Pest Management.

Jones, M. (Ed.). (1993). *Collection conservation treatment: A resource manual for program development and conservation technician training.* Berkeley, CA: University of California Library, Conservation Department.

Lull, W. P. (with Banks, P. N.). (1995). *Conservation environment guidelines for libraries and archives.* Ottawa, Canada: Canadian Council of Archives.

Merrill-Oldham, J., & Parisi, P. (1990). *Guide to the library binding institute standard for library binding.* Chicago: American Library Association.

Ogden, S. (Ed.). (1994). *Preservation of library and archival materials: A manual* (rev. and exp.). Andover, MA: Northeast Document Conservation Center.

Reilly, J. M. (1986). *Care and identification of 19th century photographic prints.* Rochester, NY: Eastman Kodak.

Swartzburg, S. G., Bussey, H., & Garretson, F. (1991). *Libraries and archives: Design and renovation with a preservation perspective.* Metuchen, NJ: Scarecrow Press.

Wilhelm, H. (1993). *The permanence and care of color photographs: Traditional and digital color prints, color negatives, slides, and motion pictures.* Grinnell, IA: Preservation.

SUGGESTED READINGS

DeBakey, L., & DeBakey, S. (1989). Our silent enemy: Ashes in our libraries. *Bulletin of the Medical Library Association, 77,* 258–268.

Kirkpatrick, B. A. (1989). Preservation activities and needs in U.S. biomedical libraries: A status report. *Bulletin of the Medical Library Association, 77,* 276–283.

Paulson, B. A. (1989). Developing a preservation policy and procedure statement for a health sciences library. *Bulletin of the Medical Library Association, 77,* 293–298.

9

Learning Resource Centers, Computer Laboratories, and Clinical Simulation Laboratories

Craig Locatis, PhD
Michael Weisberg, EdD
Debra L. Spunt, MS, RN

This chapter has three themes. The first is that the functions performed by learning resource centers (LRCs), computer laboratories (CLs), and clinical simulation laboratories (CSLs) have become vital to nursing and other health professions education due, in part, to new teaching-learning paradigms. The second theme is that information technologies are changing rapidly. These changes are transforming the nature of learning resource centers and teaching laboratories, their intraorganizational and interinstitutional relationships, and the general health professions education enterprise. The final theme is that although learning centers and teaching labs are undergoing major transformation, their basic goals are not. These goals include: making information resources available to faculty and students; providing consultation and training to enable faculty and students to use these resources effectively; and nurturing a supportive environment where faculty and students can interact with resources and each other for personal growth and development.

This chapter has four parts. The first reviews the shifting paradigms in health professions education and other forces that are significantly altering the role and importance of learning centers and teaching labs in nursing and other health professions schools. The second examines the technological trends transforming these centers and labs. The third reviews some basic practices and issues regarding application and management of technology in LRCs and CLs, while the fourth focuses on CSLs.

FACTORS INFLUENCING TECHNOLOGY/ LEARNING RESOURCE ROLES

The prevalence of information technology in health professions practice, the impact of health care reform, and changing educational paradigms suggest more central roles for learning resource centers, computer labs, and clinical simulation labs.

Information technologies are causing enormous changes in the way people entertain themselves, learn, and work (Weisberg & Ullmer, 1995). These changes result, in part, from the automation of many repetitive, mundane, or dangerous tasks, and the use of computers to augment human performance (Landauer, 1995). One or two decades ago, most information was stored in nonelectronic form, and the information that was stored on computers usually had to be entered with clerical assistance. Today, emerging digital technologies, the use of computerized patient record systems (CPRS), and the integration of patient databases with other medical systems is making it imperative that health professionals interact with information technology directly. Multimedia instruction in nursing, previously provided by slides and other traditional audiovisual media, is now primarily offered through computer-based technologies (Gleydura, Michelman, & Wilson, 1995). As early as 1986, computer-based learning resources were in use by almost half of the baccalaureate nursing programs in the United States (Hebda, 1988). Computers are being used more often in education and in clinical practice; and the explosion of biomedical knowledge has made information technology indispensable. Students and practitioners need to know not only how to use these technologies to provide clinical care, but also how to use them as electronic performance support systems (EPSs) and tools for lifelong learning.

Health care reform is altering the nature of clinical practice and the allocation of human and technology resources in medical centers and health professions schools. These changes reverberate into the health professions curricula. Since there are no more capitation grants to underwrite education costs, these expenses often have to be subsidized with clinical revenue. Health care reform's focus on cost containment increases pressure on faculty to spend more time in the direct provision of care and less time teaching. Consequently, the capacity to automate certain tasks via information technology is viewed as a way to free up faculty resources and leverage the curriculum. By using the technology to instruct at a distance, preservice and continuing education offered on-site can be provided to new and potentially larger learner populations.

Research shows students learn more in less time with computer-based instruction than with conventional classroom approaches (Belfry & Winne, 1988), thus traditional teaching strategies are changing as computers penetrate the classroom. This paradigm shift from a teacher-centered approach to a learner-centered approach demands using information technology and learning resources in new, challenging ways. This shift is known widely in the health professions as problem-based learning (Reinhardt, 1995; Twigg, 1994). Health care reform is promoting the use of technology in education for more efficiency, while the shifting paradigm is encouraging its use for greater effectiveness. The basic assumption is that students learn more effectively by assuming more responsibility for their own achievement; that is, being less dependent on their teachers. The effects of this shift on the roles of learning resource centers and teaching labs are subtle; it does *not* dictate that information technology be used as a substitute for teachers or employed only for individualized instruction.

LEARNER-CENTERED EDUCATION, INFORMATION TECHNOLOGY, AND LEARNING RESOURCES

The learner-centered, problem-based learning paradigm emphasizes active student participation in meaningful contexts over passive assimilation of abstract knowledge in traditional lecture and classroom settings. It focuses on acquiring problem-solving skills and "learning how to learn" as much as it does on acquisition of knowledge. In problem-based curricula, faculty members assume roles as facilitators and mentors, in addition to their more traditional role of imparting information. Students are encouraged to use knowledge resources and tools and to work both independently and in teams. This process enables learners to: acquire knowledge and problem-solving skills transferable to professional practice; experience the benefits of collaboration; and develop autonomous learning skills necessary for lifelong learning.

The learner-centered paradigm is based more on cognitive approaches to learning psychology in which ends and means are inseparable. In contrast, the older, behavioral approaches to learning made sharp distinctions between the objectives and methods of instruction, whereby the teacher first set educational aims and then chose the best means to achieve them. Too often this led to emphasizing efficient content acquisition over effective cognitive processing and the development of appropriate attitudes and interpersonal skills. An objective such as understanding human gross anatomy, for example, was often achieved by exposing students to slide-tape programs defining organ functions and then following up quickly with tests. Problem-solving skills, learning how to learn, learning to cooperate, and learning to function independently suffered accordingly. In contrast, with the new problem-based learning paradigm, students might study anatomy in teams, taking turns teaching each other, all within the "real-world" context of solving clinical cases.

In the new paradigm, student use of information technology and resources for both independent and cooperative learning becomes paramount (Rohfeld & Hiemstra, 1995; Locates, 1989). Rather than simply providing support, learning resource centers and teaching labs may play key roles in the curriculum (Kanter, 1995; Miller & Wolf, 1995). In fact, it can be claimed that the technologies and resources in these centers and labs, and the faculty that use them, *are* the curriculum.

TECHNOLOGY TRENDS AND IMPLICATIONS

In particular, three computing technology trends are greatly changing the nature of learning resource centers and laboratories: capacity, connectivity, and convergence. These trends are eroding the differences between traditional LRC/teaching labs and other library/information services. Computing capacity increases, while costs decline. If there is a lawfulness to advances in computing technology, it is "better, smaller, cheaper." A retrospective analysis of computer technology found that processing capacity, in terms of integrated circuits per chip, doubles about every 18 months (Gilder, 1994). This phenomenon, known as Moore's Law, has occurred without doubling the size of machines. In fact, as power has increased, size has diminished, and machines have become more portable. Increasing bandwidth, or the amount of information that can be processed in a given unit of time, is endemic not only to computers, but to a host of peripheral devices and related telecommunication technologies. As computers become increasingly integrated with other electronic devices and more popular as consumer appliances, their costs continue to drop, and these economies of scale make them more affordable for education.

Before the introduction of the microcomputer, computers were large, clumsy, complicated mainframes necessarily under specialists' control. Microcomputers, or personal computers, made the technology simpler and available to the masses. But when the technology moved from the computing center to the desktop, connectivity and communication abated. More recently, stand-alone systems were linked into local area networks (LANs) so they could share e-mail, database, and other common communication and information resources. The trend today is internetworking, or connecting local networks to form wider ones.

While some wide area networks (WANs) exist that are based on older network configurations (where individual users communicate via a single large mainframe or hub), the technology that predominates today, and the one that is used on the Internet, allows a complement of computers, both large and small, on many different, interconnected, independent networks to exchange information and communicate worldwide (Wladawsky-Berger, 1997). Instead of a single hub, multiple servers are accessed by clients. An addressing scheme and intervening telecommunications systems help ensure that information is routed appropriately. Intranets use this same publicly shared information superhighway for private purposes. Encryption, firewalls, and other security mechanisms enable only certain users to access information. The data exchanged over local and wide area networks are not just text or characters, but images, sound, and video files in formats that can be presented on different platforms. As bandwidth increases, digital multimedia files that previously could be displayed only on fast desktop computers can now be transmitted compatibly across a variety of platforms.

Convergence is the tendency toward technology integration. Diverse technologies come together or are replaced by new ones combining their separate affordances and features (Gilder, 1994; Norman, 1993). Traditional learning resource center collections of slides, audio, and video recordings in analog format are being replaced by digital technologies. Whereas previous definitions of multimedia referred to programs using combinations of text, images, audio, video, and animation, more recent definitions also stipulate these program elements should be in a digital format (Nicholls & Ridley, 1996). While more mature optical multimedia technology like the videodisc retains information in an analog format that involves using videodisc players as computer peripherals, newer optical media such as the compact disc do not. Digital compact discs include CD-ROMs for computers as well as digital audio and digital videodiscs (DVDs). Since the technologies are digital, the information they provide is more easily integrated into computing systems and delivered over computer networks. The latest methods for radio and television broadcasts are also digital. Cameras, scanners, and video boards that can capture primary information digitally are now employed. Today, the major technologies of computing, television, and telephony are coming together because of the transformation to digital information.

Convergence is occurring not only in hardware, but in software and applications. For example, programs that originally were designed for distinctive tasks, such as word processing and desktop publishing, have incorporated each other's features. Where it used to be very difficult to use resources created with one software tool with another software tool, it is now simplified. Such data exchange is done at the level of the computer's operating system, so no file conversion is necessary as long as the applications run on the same platform. Moreover, it is possible to emulate different computer operating systems, and the intervening emulation can be used to run applications designed for different platforms. Software-only solutions for presenting networked multimedia—such as those associated with client/server technology, markup languages like the HyperText Markup Language (HTML), and virtual machines and programming languages like Java allow cross-platform compatibility and resource sharing on the Internet and within intranets (Juliussen, 1997).

Formerly, computer-based training programs were "uncoupled" from the actual content, systems, or devices that they were developed to teach, even when programs taught computer applications. But since more jobs today involve competency using computers or devices linked to them, it is possible to create computer-based instruction programs that embed training within the products and applications people must learn. The training can be just-in-time and on-demand; that is, evoked by users on the job at the moment they need it (Winslow & Bramer, 1994). In addition, it is possible to provide online help, job aids, reference works, expert consultation systems, databases, and other forms of electronic performance support (Gery, 1991). Such training technology convergence may even involve designing user interfaces that are so intuitive and self-explanatory that no instruction is needed. The differences between information systems and training systems are eroded when both online documentation and tutorials become embedded in computer applications that support work (Locatis, 1989).

279

The implications of these trends for learning resource centers and teaching laboratories are clear. First, modern resource centers and teaching labs should be integrated, both physically and functionally with each another and with other information resources in health professions schools (Nowacek & Friedman, 1995). As technologies converge, so will heretofore separate library, learning resource center and computer lab functions (Schmidt & Mitchell, 1994). Second, resource centers and labs should be linked to other computing resources inside and outside the academic institution. Libraries and learning resource centers of the future will be "virtual," comprising online information residing on many different servers (Locatis & Weisberg, in press) accessible from wherever learners are located. Third, the online, electronic information resources will include new data forms. As computing technology begins to accommodate three-dimensional and other types of information, computer-based simulation devices incorporating tactile response and immersive virtual reality displays will become more prevalent. The National Library of Medicine's Visible Human Project has already stored complete adult male and female anatomy in a computer (Spitzer, Ackerman, Scherzinger, & Whitlock, 1996). Primary information, such as that comprising the Visible Humans data set, will become more common online. These data sets and virtual reality databases will take their place alongside more traditional information resources in libraries and learning resource centers. While LRCs and CLs will be affected most immediately by technology trends, CSLs also will be impacted.

GENERAL POLICIES, PRACTICES, AND ISSUES

Several general policies, practices, and issues affect the relationships among learning resource centers, computer labs, and clinical simulation labs as well as their roles within the academic community. The managers of these resources should work with others within the academic institution to shape organizational computing and information policies and to ensure the effective integration of learning resources into the curriculum. They should participate in the decision making that impacts both the curriculum and the use of computing/information technology. This involvement should be at all levels—within the health professions department and school, within the academic medical center, and when appropriate, within the university. LRCs and CLs should be part of the library, if a nursing school has one. If not, an attempt should be made to coordinate its functions with those of the general health science or academic library and to draw on the resources and expertise of the library and related information and media services, such as those of the computing and biomedical communications centers.

A paramount issue is the functional relationships among the LRC, CL, and CSL. While each of these units may function separately, it is probably more efficient to manage them as a single unit. Depending on the size of a program, a single learning resource director might manage all three; or each might have individual directors who report to the person responsible for all information resources within the institution, including those in libraries and computing centers. In any event, an attempt should be made to locate these units together to capitalize on the technology and to use staff more effectively and efficiently. Contiguous location also enables using the computer lab as a classroom when LRC staff teach computer and online information systems to users or when faculty want to bring classes to the LRC to use computer-based learning and applications software.

The CL can be used to teach classes on e-mail, database, and Internet accessible information resources as well as the use of word processing, spreadsheet, graphics, multimedia authoring, and other software. At other times, it can be a lab in which students use these programs to complete projects and assignments. Whether a computer lab also can function as a classroom depends on the faculty. If classroom use of computers and multimedia resources is substantial, it is preferable to have a separate multimedia classroom.

The learning resource center and computing lab should be part of an integrated on-site/off-site academic information system providing electronic mail, online catalog, and other services (Schmidt & Mitchell, 1994). LRCs and CLs should have their own local

281

area networks connected to an institutional or campuswide network and to the Internet. Faculty should be able to access these networks from their offices, and students living on-site should be able to access them from their living quarters. Offices, dormitories, wards, and clinics should be interconnected, and the connectivity should extend off-site, so that faculty and students can access the network from work and home. Practitioners enrolled in continuing education programs and others involved in distance-learning programs should have access to the same services as those on-site. The use of client/server computing technology and the Internet should be encouraged to provide access; and the technology should be leveraged, when appropriate, by creating a private intranet accessible only to qualified users.

Efforts should be made to foster student and faculty "use" of computing technology. Student ownership of computers might be mandated and included in the costs of tuition. Another approach is to offer loans, discounts, and other incentives. Computing technology should be provided to staff in the workplace. They also might be offered purchasing incentives, or be loaned older, surplus equipment for home use. Free e-mail accounts and information services should be provided or at least be made available at the lowest possible cost.

A general policy regarding computing technology should be developed. One issue is whether the institution should support a single computer and/or operating system or multiple ones. In any event, the use of hardware and software that enables resource sharing among applications and interoperability among platforms should be encouraged. Preference should be given to systems and software that most easily allow file sharing over networks. The acquisition of machines with network adapter cards, modems, and other telecommunication technology that employ client/server software should be encouraged.

LRC/CL POLICIES, PRACTICES, AND ISSUES

Most of the policies, practices, and issues related to the specific functions of learning resource centers and computer labs fall into three broad areas: space allocation, hardware/software acquisition and use, and resource management.

Space and Furniture

The LRC and CL design should follow sound ergonomic principles (Harwin & Haynes, 1992; Pascarelli & Quilter, 1994; Sellers, 1994; Weisberg, 1993). Space should be sufficient to accommodate the collection and the anticipated number of users during peak time periods. Space requirements will depend on factors such as the magnitude of the academic program, the size of the student body, the number of computer-related course offerings, and the degree to which faculty provide individualized instruction and incorporate electronic learning resources into their courses.

There should be public and private areas for housing the collection, for storing materials and equipment, and for faculty and student use. If faculty and students want to create their own materials, and there is no biomedical communications department providing these services already, than space should be allotted for slide and document scanning, digitizing, and editing video, and for the use of graphics software and authoring tools. Some of these resources might be placed in the computer lab.

Tables and carrels should be set up in LRC public areas for individual use of video cassettes and interactive multimedia technology; the equipment in these areas should be equipped with headsets to control acoustics. There also should be small, private study rooms with whiteboards and interactive multimedia and videocassette devices for group use. Since problem-based curricula encourage students to work together, a space should be provided where they can interact with the technology and with each other in small groups without disrupting other LRC users.

A computer lab must be secure, accessible after hours, and staffed by persons providing technical assistance. Consequently, locating it within the LRC is not only convenient, it enables the same staff to supervise both areas. The lab can occupy a separate room inside the LRC; a glass wall can be erected to control acoustics while allowing for visual monitoring of the area. Curtains can be drawn to isolate the area when needed and to control light. It is important that the computer lab have its own electrical circuits as well as independent lighting and climate controls. In addition, higher levels of ventilation and cooling will be necessary, since there will be times when all the machines will be in use and the lab will be crowded.

The LRC and CL should have sectional lighting with rheostats installed. A master control should be conveniently located behind the service desk in the LRC for regulating all lighting. In the CL, lighting controls should be located in front, near an instructor workstation. A projection screen should also be set up in front, and it should be possible to darken that part of the room. The screen should be sheltered from glare and all external light sources, such as windows. Ideally, the lab will have a high ceiling for mounting a video projector. If not, portable projectors can be used.

Adjustable chairs at least 15 to 17 inches deep and at least 18 inches wide, and long flat desks least 30 inches deep and 48 inches wide are recommended (Weisberg, 1993). Tables might be preferable to carrels, even in the LRC's individual study areas, because so much of the carrel work area is usually consumed by the equipment, leaving insufficient space for note-taking and other student activities. Tables also make it easier for two or three students to work together; and when classes are held in the computer lab, students may need to share machines. Computer tables should be between 23 and 28.5 inches high (lower than standard ones), and adjustable, to accommodate typing and keyboarding at an appropriate angle (Weisberg, 1993). If tables with these lower heights are not available, retractable trays or keying surfaces attached below the work surface can be installed.

Ideally, tables will come with built-in shelving so that computers, peripherals, and other materials can be placed underneath, but within easy reach. Tables should be wide enough so that all equipment can rest on the desktop. In the CL, tables should be wide enough to accommodate monitor placement alongside the computers, not on top, which not only reduces comfort, but may obstruct the view of projected material. The preferred monitor viewing angle is 10 to 20 degrees below horizontal; and to prevent glare, tables should be placed so that monitors can be set at 90-degree angles to windows and never directly in front of windows (Weisberg, 1993).

Multiple outlets or power strips should be installed along each wall in the LRC and the CL. A false floor in the CL and possibly in the individual and group study areas of the LRC is also a possibility, permitting wiring and cabling to be run under the floor to workstations in the center of the room. This precludes disconnections and damage to cabling and is safer for users. If false floors are installed, the ideal are those made with removable carpet tiles, for acoustical purposes and for easy removal to access wiring. There should be higher ceilings in false-floor areas to compensate for the loss of airspace. More space will be needed at the entrances to these areas to accommodate ramps for handicapped access.

Finally, if possible, the computer lab also should have special switching technology that can be controlled from the instructor workstation. This technology should be capable of directing output from any workstation to all the other workstations and to the projector. Such a device ensures unobstructed display at each desktop. It is also useful for directing student attention because it can be used to temporarily lock students out of their keyboards.

Hardware/Software

Obviously, computing, multimedia, and other hardware and software, including network technology, must be acquired for both the LRC and CL, which should be part of campus or institutional cable and computer networks with Internet access. If the institution is actively involved in distance learning and/or providing services via the Internet, the LRC may need its own Web server or have a presence on some other institutional server that Internet users can access. Any new cabling should support the maximum available bandwidth, and it should be installed so that it can be replaced and upgraded in the future. Local area network technology can be used to back up systems in the CL and LRC, although a special dedicated server with a data tape drive will be necessary for this purpose. CD-ROM servers and other servers can be placed online and used to deliver multimedia and applications software over networks (Wolfe, 1994).

Any multimedia computing hardware should accommodate course materials and programs and/or commercial products readily available in the marketplace. When purchasing hardware, product directories (such as the one published by the International Communications Industries Association) and individual manufacturer and supplier catalogs should be consulted. Computers should be compatible and interoperable with other systems used within the institution. In general, multimedia computers should have multisync displays, speakers, CD-ROM drives, and the highest-speed processors available, largest-capacity hard disks, and as much general and video RAM as possible. Multimedia programs are bandwidth-intensive, therefore both the computers and the networks connecting them should provide the maximum amount of bandwidth an institution can afford.

Videodisc players may be desirable as well, although this older, interactive analog television technology is being usurped by compact disc, digital videodisc, and network technologies employing digital multimedia. There are, however, many high-quality videodisc programs and some minimal investment in the format may be warranted (Locatis, 1995). Of course, videocassette players, slide projectors, overhead projectors, and audiocassette players still will be needed to accommodate these other media formats. Portable screens, extension cords, power strips, and additional cables and projection bulbs also should be readily available.

A sufficient number of machines must be installed to accommodate students in the computer lab and the LRC's individual study areas at peak times. Machines also should be provided in small group study areas. Multimedia computing systems, videocassette players, and video projectors should be placed on portable carts if permanent machines cannot be installed. These "portable workstations" can be moved to small group study areas, or loaned for classroom use, if the LRC is responsible for classroom audiovisual services. They also can be used for backup when other systems malfunction. Depending on institutional policy and budget, laptop machines might be made available to faculty and/or students for short-term loan.

Video projectors should support both television and computer output, and multiple computer display resolutions should be accommodated. The projectors should have sufficient luminance to display in lighted environments and adjustable lenses to allow for large-image displays at short distances from the screen, since most projection will likely be from instructor workstations or desks at the front of a room. In addition, the projectors should have built-in speakers and amplifiers, enabling display of both images and sounds without relying on external audio equipment.

Software and online services should reflect the needs of the academic program and be compatible with the delivery platforms available. In addition to multimedia, general applications software such as spreadsheet, word processing, and graphics programs might be made available, as well as special applications software for modeling and statistical analysis. Online resources should also be identified, such as multimedia programs and information resources accessible via the World Wide Web. Some general directories to multimedia programs include: *CD-ROMs in Print,* from Gale Research, and the *Multimedia and Videodisc Compendium,* from Emerging Technology Consultants. Key directory and catalog sources to multimedia programs more specific to nursing include: the *Directory of Educational Software for Nursing* published by FITNE, Incorporated; the *Interactive Healthcare Videodisc Directory,* the *Interactive Healthcare CD-ROM Directory,* and the *Interactive Healthcare CAI Directory,* published by Stewart Publishing; and the catalog of Lippincott-Raven Publishers. Online sources to nursing materials include the National Library of Medicine AVLINE database on audiovisuals, and *Software for Health Sciences Education: A Resource Catalog,* a database distributed by the University of Michigan. Product reviews appear regularly in newsletters and journals, such as the *Interactive Healthcare Newsletter* by Stewart Publishing and *Computers in Nursing* by Lippincott-Raven. In addition, journals occasionally publish bibliographies of health care information resources (cf. Interagency Council on Information Resources for Nursing, 1996).

While individual faculty may identify resources to include in the LRC collection, it also is useful to have a selection committee composed of faculty and students to aid in this purpose (Van Ort, 1989). The committee can be used to develop collection policies and courseware evaluation procedures, and to assess the center's core collection to ensure that it is balanced to reflect the entire curriculum. Forms, checklists, and faculty development seminars can be employed to help instructors make better judgments about courseware and other materials. These tools should focus faculty attention on valid selection criteria (Van Ort, 1989). The programs should be compatible with available hardware, teach valid content using appropriate instructional strategies, and have a user interface that is easy and intuitive. They also should provide indexes, searching capabilities, and other online information resources and retrieval aids conducive to self-directed learning (Nicholls & Ridley, 1996).

For all programs and applications, original copies of videocassette and floppy disks should be kept as backup; or additional copies of nonrecordable programs on videodisc or CD-ROM should be acquired. If extra copies are not maintained, use will have to be monitored closely. A better option, though, is to make them network accessible, which is possible since programs on CD-ROMs and floppy disks use digital information. Other advantages to this alternative are that fewer copies would be needed, and resource management and tracking could be automated. However, to implement this option networked versions of the software must be acquired so that it can be used simultaneously (Wolfe, 1994).

Management

Professional and paraprofessional staff must have appropriate technical expertise; and policies and procedures must establish operating hours, access, scheduling, hardware/software use, and loans. In addition, materials and equipment must be cataloged and inventoried, and their use documented and assessed. Finally, strategies for faculty/student development must be defined. A written policy should cover such vital issues as appropriate use, user responsibilities, sanctions for misuse, privacy, copyright, costs, security, and public access to resources and services. It is imperative that both staff and users be informed of policies, and that policies be consistently enforced.

The number and type of staff to hire depends on the magnitude of operations. At least one person on staff should have both general library-media and computing technology skills. Subspecialists may need to be hired, unless those working in other institutional units can be utilized on a cooperative basis. For example, instead of hiring a cataloger or network specialist, it might be possible to use the cataloging services of the library or network services of the computing center. A policy may be needed to define which, if any, services will be available to outsiders or the general public, including online and/or Internet-accessible resources. Schedules must structure class use of the computer lab, group use of study rooms, and perhaps, student use of individual equipment. The LRC should be open after hours and on weekends. Sufficient safeguards should be established to protect copyrighted software.

Users need to be able to search and browse the center's collection, either in a union catalog or one specifically for the center. An inventory of all hardware and applications software must be kept up to date. It is very important to document the number of faculty and students using the lab, and the center generally, as well as specific resources and equipment. This information can be used to purge the collection and set priorities for software and hardware upgrades. It can also be used to justify programs and budget.

Workshops and seminars should be offered to familiarize faculty with the multimedia and information resources and educate them about new technology and its appropriate use; students need orientations and instruction on how to use online information sources, equipment, and applications software. Newsletters, announcements, electronic bulletin boards, Web pages, and other mechanisms should be considered as ways of meeting these obligations.

Center staff should participate on decision-making committees, attend faculty meetings, and interact with faculty members
individually to inform them about center programs, monitor their
needs, and obtain continuous feedback. In addition, periodic surveys should be conducted to determine faculty/student satisfaction and service requirements. Surveys should evaluate the extent
to which different services are used, the quality of the services,
and service efficiency (Ludwig, 1993). For example, they should
ask: To what extent do faculty members use the LRC for classroom activities and/or homework assignments? To what extent do
they use existing resources versus developing their own? Are they
satisfied with the services staff provide? Is the turnaround time
acceptable for staff provided services, such as interlibrary loans,
software acquisition and media production?

CLINICAL SIMULATION LABORATORIES

The exponential increase in information, rapidly evolving technology, and changes in the health care environment have facilitated the
increasing need for Clinical Simulation Laboratories (CSL). Today's
CSLs are found not only in schools of nursing but also in hospitals,
home health care agencies, and long-term care facilities. These CSLs
can promote and support a variety of teaching strategies while
preparing an active participant in the process of lifelong learning.

The primary purpose of the clinical simulation laboratory is
to replicate the essential aspects of a clinical situation and/or environment so that the same or similar situation may be understood and managed in any type of clinical practice setting
(Hanson, 1993). The laboratory experience expands, reinforces,
and applies the knowledge acquired in the classroom and learning
resource/media center. Clinical simulation helps the learner to
develop critical thinking skills and focus on psychomotor skill
development without the environmental distractions often found
in the patient care setting (McKeachie, 1994). The CSL facilitates the active learning of new skills, review and refinement of
old skills, and the introduction of new technology (equipment).
The simulation experience provides the student and health care

professional with immediate feedback and reinforcement of learning (Roberts, While, & Fitzpatrick, 1992).

Components of the Clinical Simulation Laboratory

The clinical simulation laboratories of today and the future must be able to replicate multiple clinical settings and situations. Unlike the direct patient care approach to clinical instruction, the CSL offers a controlled, dependable, consistent, and structured learning setting (Alspach, 1995). The learning laboratory provides a supportive atmosphere that serves as a catalyst in the applied learning process. The key to this is organization, flexibility of the environment, technology support, and equipment.

Space. The allocation of space reflects the agency/institutional commitment and needs. Several key components need to be considered when designing a CSL facility to make it functional and at the same time flexible. The laboratory's physical environment should lend itself to multiple teaching strategies; for example, teacher-directed (formal demonstration, return demonstration), small group, and self-directed learning. The identification of potential teaching approaches to be used will determine the exact needs of each laboratory (deTournyay & Thompson, 1987).

After the teaching strategies have been identified, the design phase of laboratory development can begin. The actual space selection is dependent on the predicted utilization and room availability. The laboratory may be in an out-of-service (unused) hospital room (if the CSL is part of a clinical agency) a classroom, or a room with the LRC. Regardless of the type of laboratory or space limitations, however, a few basic items need to be considered when selecting the appropriate space. All laboratories must have good ventilation and illumination, a sink, ample electrical outlets and storage space, and a security system. Access to the agency's computer systems and any computerized educational simulation programs should be included in space and laboratory design.

The actual laboratory design can be as basic as a bed and overbed table or as complex as a fully functional critical care unit with monitors, suction, and power columns. On the average, a teaching unit or bed station should be large enough to allow up to six students to work together. If the laboratory will be used for teaching physical assessment where student or professional models serve as the patients, the space needs to include ceiling tracks appropriate for the installation of privacy curtains. Additional space modifications may be required based on the intended use of the CSL, the teaching strategy to be used, and the number of individuals using the laboratory at anytime.

Space allocation must account for storage and equipment preparation areas that are in and or immediately adjacent to the CSL. Like the individual simulation laboratories, the storage area should be well ventilated and illuminated, with electrical outlets, running water, and some type of security system. This area must be large enough for the storage of durable and disposable equipment, manikins of varying sizes and shapes, and simulators. The utilization of metal and wooden lockable cabinets will provide a safe enclosed area for the storage of disposable, electrical, and sensitive equipment. Wire, metal, or wooden shelf units, which are sturdy and have extra-wide shelves, are appropriate for the storage of manikins and simulators in individual carrying cases. In addition to storage, this area will be used for equipment repair/maintenance, and setup. A table or tabletop shelf makes an ideal work area. Plastic bins can be used to hold disposable supplies for a particular laboratory or for quick restocking, and can be stored on an open shelf.

Equipment and Simulators. The careful selection of both durable and disposable equipment will increase the ability of the institution to simulate real clinical situations. All equipment selected should be in good operating condition and reflect current technology. The use of out-of-date durable equipment makes it difficult for the learner to transfer skills and knowledge to the patient care setting. For example, an old patient-controlled analgesia pump that is no longer manufactured or used would not be appropriate for simulation. Choosing the equipment to purchase should factor in the possibility of future upgrades or the trade-in for new models. Before deciding on medical/durable equipment, the following questions should be answered:

How often and who will be using the equipment?

Will this equipment be used by a large number of clinical agencies in your area?

What is the possibility of obtaining necessary disposable equipment related to this equipment at a reduced fee or at no cost (e.g., tubing for an intravenous pump or controller)?

What is the availability of educational material for students and faculty, including in-service classes on-site?

The purchase and maintenance of medical equipment can be very expensive, labor-intensive, and require sophisticated technology. Facing the reality that most CSLs operate on a tight budget and with limited technological resources, the rental, leasing, borrowing, or sharing of equipment are all viable options that provide access to specialized equipment when needed.

Medical/Durable Equipment. Selecting state-of-the-art medical/durable equipment for purchase can be a little like buying a car, in that the same basic product is available from many, many vendors. Therefore, before purchasing equipment, it is essential to assess the equipment currently in use. Visit local health care agencies that use the equipment under consideration to observe its quality and function in a real clinical setting. Contact the agency's purchasing department for information related to the equipment. Ask for the manufacturer's/distributor's name and phone number, cost of the product, any special contractual agreement related to the equipment (e.g., free tubing), and reliability of the company. Obtain this type of information related to several vendors who sell the same equipment. Contact each vendor and competitors for information and services available with equipment purchase. When communicating with the prospective vendor emphasize the intended use of the equipment and makeup of the learners who will be using the equipment. Keep in mind that any individuals using the equipment who may have potential current and future purchasing influence may facilitate a reduction in price, a donation, and/or some type creative purchasing agreement (e.g., purchase one item at the regular price and get the second free or at a substantial reduction). After

293

reviewing all available information related to the equipment, follow your agency's policy related to procurement of durable equipment. Keep copies of all ordering and purchasing requisitions to help track purchasing requests and vendors. Upon delivery of the equipment, immediately test it. If possible, coordinate the delivery and testing of the equipment with the vendor for an in-service session on the operation of the equipment.

Disposable Equipment. The medical equipment selected will become the frame of the laboratory, and the disposable equipment will be the component related to the daily operation of the facility. The identification of quantity and type of disposable equipment will be dependent on the number of learners and types of laboratory experience (e.g., open laboratory that allows for unlimited repeated practice, structured laboratory with limited practice, or competency validation or testing). Equipment can be purchased through medical supply companies or directly from a clinical agency. It is often slightly more economical to arrange for an ongoing purchase agreement with a local hospital and to buy items in bulk. Purchasing agreements should include the delivery and replacement of damaged goods by the vendor or hospital. Upon delivery, the supplies should be cataloged and shelved in a clean dry area located in or adjacent to the CSL.

A cost-saving alternative to new disposable equipment is to use of out-of-date supplies and medications. This will make it possible to increase the quantity of available practice supplies without increased cost, thus ensuring that learners have access to equipment currently being used in health care agencies. In simulation, sterile supplies are not used on actual wounds and medications/intravenous fluids are not administered to live people. Thus, the use of out-of-date disposable equipment and medications will enhance learning and cause no harm.

Manikins, Models, and Simulators. The final, and possibly the most important supplies in the CSL are the manikins, models, and clinical simulators. The use of clinical simulators in a well-stocked laboratory allows for the transformation of a plain room into a clinical environment. Lifelike manikins, anatomical models, and simulators facilitate the assessment, problem-solving, critical-thinking process in conjunction with psychomotor skill development necessary to prepare students and health care providers to deliver safe and efficient patient care in multiple health care arenas (home, hospital, long-term care, school, business). Manikins and clinical simulators can be tailored to meet individual student needs and teaching strategies.

Keeping in mind that the primary goal of the CSL is to replicate or closely approximate reality, the faculty or laboratory coordinator will identify which skills will be simulated using peers and which ones will be simulated on manikins. Lifelike manikins that can assume different positions will enhance teaching strategies and test methods. As with medical equipment, multiple vendors manufacture and market manikins for the health care professional. Before purchase, the factors to evaluate include durability, repair/maintenance requirements, parts replacement, and storage requirements.

The "skin" of manikins is made of vinyl, flexible or rigid plastic, and fabric. It must be able to tolerate repeated applications of chemicals such as betadine and tincture of benzoin, and be easy to clean with soap and water. Dressing-change, incision, and other manikins will require cleaning with an adhesive remover. Movable parts and limbs are constructed of hard plastic and a type of metal, and are attached with hinges and/or a type of bolt and nut device. In addition to moveable external parts, some manikins—such as the one used for assessment of the prostate gland—have interchangeable internal parts, which often slide into place via a track and are secured in place with a nut and bolt.

The repair/maintenance and parts replacement of manikins will depend on the frequency of use, number and type of moving parts, and the type of simulation skills to be performed. For example, manikins used for catheterization and rectal examination may become torn or cracked as a result of frequent internal manipulation. Glue (for vinyl and plastic), sutures, and hot pen (used to soften an area to be remolded and or fused) can be used to repair and reinforce weak or high-stress areas. Replacement parts are often included with the manikin or available for purchase. Skin and veins can be easily replaced on those used for psychomotor skills training related to intravenous therapy. Usually, when manikin parts are irreparably broken, and replacement parts are no longer available, it is possible to interchange parts among manikins or modify the intended use of the "disabled" manikin based on its limitation/capabilities. For example, a manikin whose legs have been destroyed can be treated as a bilateral amputee, used for tracheostomy care, enteral feedings, and other skills simulation, which do not involve the lower limbs.

Manikins, although expensive, usually will last a long time with proper care, preventive maintenance, and proper storage. Most manufacturers provide a storage unit for each manikin at the time of purchase, commonly a soft leather zipper bag with carrying strap, a canvas zipper bag with cloth handles, a nylon zipper bag with cloth handles, a Ziploctype plastic bag, a cardboard box with attached or detachable lid, hard plastic box, or hard-sided case. Storage areas must be dry and cool; extremes of hot and dry may cause the mannequins' external internal and external parts to be come fragile, cracked, and more prone to damage. Mildew, mold, spores, and bacteria may grow on and in manikins that are not cleaned and thoroughly dried before storage, or that become wet/damp in the storage area.

Today's practitioners must be able to provide high-quality care to a more diverse population, thus the development of clinical/assessment simulators for use in the CSL is ongoing. These simulators add to the ability of the CSL to replicate myriad clinical situations, and emphasize critical thinking and prioritization skills needed for decision making and safe clinical practice. The most realistic and advanced simulators are those related to normal and abnormal health-assessment findings (eye, ear, heart and lung sounds, and reproductive organs) and cardiovascular interpretation. Health-assessment simulators can be used by learners at all levels. The beginning nursing student can learn basic assessment skills and to differentiate normal and abnormal findings. The nurse practitioner can use the data assessed via the simulator to determine a differential diagnosis and appropriate medical/nursing treatment to be prescribed. Simulators used in the area of cardiovascular nursing range from arrhythmia/dysrhythmia interpretation, hemodynamic monitoring, to the integration of multiple simulators for the purpose of "mock codes."

Scheduling, Inventory, and Restocking

The day-to-day functions of the CSL depend on a preplanned organized scheduling and supply distribution and replenishment system. In an ideal world, CSL utilization would make it possible to predict schedule and supply needs prior to the start of the academic year. But extra classes, additional student needs, tours, and presentations for community groups are some of the indeterminates that may pop up at the last minute. Nevertheless, for the most part, it is possible to predict with some degree of accuracy the needs of an academic unit on a per-semester basis.

Recordkeeping is the key component to organization and smooth operation in the CSL. It should include room schedules, student data, supplies needed and supplies used, indicators related to supply/equipment replacement, and any additional data specific to your CSL. The CSL documentation process may be a paper-and-pencil system, automated, or a combination, based on the size of the CSL and computer access.

Scheduling. A general request for scheduling should be submitted a semester or six months in advance of the beginning of the academic semester or unit for which the laboratories will be used. The faculty coordinating or in charge of the courses requiring laboratory time should communicate the following information to the CSL manager:

Course number and title.

Faculty responsible for laboratory portion of course.

Phone/beeper numbers and e-mail addresses of faculty.

Date of request (to help prioritize room assignments).

Day of week, time of day, and dates laboratory will be needed.

Number of students.

Purpose of laboratory and any special needs (AV, ventilator, crash cart, simulators).

Detailed list or description of what will be taught in each laboratory session (for laboratory setup).

The laboratory reservation may be made in writing or via electronic mail.

Inventory and Restocking. The volumes of equipment, supplies, and transactions which are needed for the day-to-day operation of a CSL with limited staff and resources necessitates a structured record-keeping program. The inventory system can be written or automated. The selection or development of an automated record-keeping system for the CSL has been found to save time and increase accuracy related to supply distribution and acquisition. A system should provide cross-referencing (skills to be taught with equipment and supplies needs), automatic notification of low inventory items, notification related to routine equipment maintenance/calibration, and have the ability to generate reports (Hodson et al., 1988). No matter what format is selected, one must be able to retrieve information related to equipment, manikins, models, simulators, supplies set up for a laboratory section or unit, supplies actually used, and quantity available in storage.

Although durable equipment, manikins, models, and simulators do not to need to be replaced on a regular basis, records of their use must be kept current to ensure they are in working order. The inventory format related to equipment should include: type of equipment (beds, power columns), manufacturer information (name, vendor, phone numbers), serial number, cost, and location in CSL. The consolidation of information facilitates quick access on data for repair, education, and checking for replacement by newly released equipment from a particular manufacturer.

Keeping track of disposable supplies to be used, and those actually used, can be one of the most difficult, time consuming aspect related to the functioning of the CSL. The inventory of this equipment can either be formatted by skill to be used for (tracheostomy care), by the type of equipment (sterile gauze pads 2x2s, 4x4s) or cross references which allows one to change the format based on the need at the time (i.e., laboratory set up or review of total equipment per category available). An inventory system spread sheet should contain the item name, description, location in CSL, cost and how available for purchase (individual, box, case), and where and how to order supplies (hospital central supply, supply vendor) for the CSL (Reimer, 1992). The system should also be able to provide an accurate inventory of supplies on hand, thus eliminating the labor intensive process of counting every item at the end of a semester prior to ordering.

Clinical simulation laboratories are a major component of most schools of nursing curricula, but they are very costly to run, a major concern in these days of tight budgets and budget cuts. Therefore, careful planning and organization of space, equipment, manikins, models, simulators, and supplies will facilitate the smooth and cost-effective functioning of a laboratory facility. Today's CSL can closely replicate the clinical environment and prepare students to provide safe, individualized care.

CONCLUSION

An assumption underlying this chapter is that libraries, learning resource centers, and teaching laboratories will become virtual as the boundaries between academic institutions and the outside world disappear. Therefore it has stressed building physical infrastructures, such as networks, and creating appropriate organizational interrelationships that can accommodate this change. As technology trends of computing capacity, connectivity, and convergence continue to evolve, it is safe to assume that learning resource centers, computer laboratories, and clinical simulation laboratories will eventually become seamlessly linked both inside and outside the institution.

REFERENCES

Alspach, J. G. (1995). *The educational process in nursing staff development.* St. Louis, MO: Mosby Yearbook.

Belfry, M., & Winne, P. (1988). A review of the effectiveness of computer-assisted instruction in nursing education. *Computers in Nursing, 6*(2), 77–85.

deTournyay, R., & Thompson, M. A. (1987). *Strategies for teaching nursing* (3rd ed.). New York: Delmar.

Gery, G. J. (1991). *Electronic performance support systems.* Boston: Weingarten.

Gilder, G. (1994). *Life after television: The coming transformation of media and American life.* New York: Norton.

Gleydura, A., Michelman, J., & Wilson, N. (1995). Multimedia training in nursing education. *Computers in Nursing, 13*(4), 169–175.

Hanson, G. F. (1993). Refocusing the skills laboratory. *Nurse Educator, 18*(2), 10–12.

Harwin, R., & Haynes, C. (1992). *Healthy computing: Risks and remedies every computer user needs to know.* New York: American Management Association.

Hebda, T. (1988). A profile of the use of computer-assisted instruction within baccalaureate nursing education. *Computer in Nursing, 6*(2), 77–85.

Hodson, K. E., Manis, J., Thayer, M., Webb, S., Hunnicutt, C., & Hoogenboom, A. (1988). Computerized management program for the skills laboratory of a school of nursing. *Computers in Nursing, 6*(5), 215–221.

Interagency Council on Information Resources for Nursing. (1996). Essential nursing references. *N&HC: Perspectives on Community, 17*(5), 255–259.

Juliussen, E. (1997, January). Technology 1997 analysis & forecast-computers. *IEEE Spectrum, 34*(1) 49–54.

Kanter, S. L. (1995, March/April). Information management of a medical school educational program: A state-of-the-art application. *Journal of the American Medical Informatics Association, 3*(2), 103–111.

Landauer, T. K. (1995). *The trouble with computers: Usefulness, usability, and productivity.* Cambridge, MA: MIT Press.

Locatis, C. (1995). Deciding among interactive multimedia technologies. *Journal of Biocommunication, 22*(2), 2–7.

Locatis, C. (1989). Information retrieval systems and learning. *Performance Improvement Quarterly, 2*(3), 4–15.

Locatis, C., & Weisberg, M. (in press). Distributed learning and the Internet. *Contemporary Education.*

Ludwig, L. (1993). Evaluating biomedical media services. *Journal of Biocommunication, 20*(3), 2–9.

McKeachie, W. J. (1994). *Teaching tips: Strategies, research, and theory* (9th ed.). Lexington, MA: D.C. Heath.

Miller, J. G., & Wolf, F. M. (1995). Strategies for integrating computer-based activities into your educational environment: A practical guide. *Journal of the American Medical Informatics Association, 3*(2), 112–117.

Nicholls, P., & Ridley, J. (1996). A context for evaluating multimedia. *Computers in Libraries, 16*(4), 34–39.

Norman, D. (1993). *Things that make us smart.* Reading, MA: Addison-Wesley.

Nowacek, G., & Friedman, C. P. (1995, December). Issues and challenges in the design of curriculum information systems. *Academic Medicine, 70*(12), 1096–1100.

Pascarelli, E., & Quilter, D. (1994). *Repetitive strain injury: A computer user's guide.* New York: Wiley.

Reimer, M. S. (1992). Computerized cost analysis for the nursing skills laboratory. *Nurse Educator, 17*(4), 8–11.

Reinhardt, A. (1995, March). New ways to learn. *BYTE, 20*(3) 50–72.

Rohfeld, R. W., & Hiemstra, R. (1995). Moderating discussions in the electronic classroom. In Z. Berge & M. Collins (Eds.), *Computer mediated communication and the online classroom: Vol. 3. Distance learning.* Cresskill, NJ: Hampton Press.

Roberts, J., While, A., & Fitzpatrick, J. (1992). Simulation: Current status in nurse education. *Nurse Education Today, 12,* 409–415.

Schmidt, D., & Mitchell, J. (1994). The J. Otto Lottes Health Sciences Library and the microcomputer laboratory. *Computer Methods and Programs in Biomedicine, 44,* 193–199.

Sellers, D. (1994). *Zap! How your computer can hurt you—and what you can do about it.* San Francisco, CA: Peachpit Press.

Spitzer, V., Ackerman, M., Scherzinger, A., & Whitlock, D. (1996). The visible human male: A technical report. *Journal of the American Medical Informatics Association, 3*(2), 118–130.

Twigg, C. (1994). The changing definition of learning. *Educom Review, 29*(4), 22–25.

Van Ort, S. (1989). Evaluating audiovisual and computer programs for classroom use. *Nurse Educator, 14*(1), 16–18.

Weisberg, M., & Ullmer, J. (1995). *Distance learning revisited. Lifelong learning and the national information infrastructure.* Proceedings of Selected Research Papers of the Association for Educational Communication and Technology (AECT), pp. 1–25. (ERIC Document Reproduction Service No. ED 383 345)

Weisberg, M. (1993). Guidelines for designing effective and healthy learning environments for interactive technologies. Interpersonal computing and technology: An electronic journal for the 21st century. ISSN 1064-4326. April, 1993 Vol. 1, No. 2. IPCT-L @GEORGETOWN EDU

Winslow, C. D., & Bramer, W. L. (1994). *Future work: Putting knowledge to work in the knowledge economy.* New York: Free Press.

Wladawsky-Berger, I. (1997). Technology 1997 analysis & forecast-viewpoint: The Internet is it. *IEEE Spectrum, 34*(1), 54.

Wolfe, J. (1994). Special considerations for networking multimedia CD-ROM titles. *CD-ROM Professional, 7*(1), 55–57.

SUGGESTED READINGS

Gomez, G. E., & Gomez, E. A. (1987). Learning of psychomotor skills: Laboratory versus patient care setting. *Journal of Nursing Education, 26,* 20–24.

Hanna, D. R. (1991). Using simulation to teach clinical nursing. *Nurse Educator, 16*(2), 28.

Hodson, K. E., Manis, J., Thayer, M., Webb, S., Hunnicutt, C., & Hoogenboom, A. (1988). Computerized management program for the skills laboratory of a school of nursing. *Computers in Nursing, 6*(5), 215–221.

Klasing, J. P. (1991). *Designing and renovating school library media centers.* Chicago: American Library Association.

Locatis, C. (1996). *An interactive multimedia technology primer.* Bethesda, MD: National Library of Medicine.

Reilly, D. E., & Oermann, M. H. (1992). *Clinical teaching in nursing education* (2nd ed.). New York: National League for Nursing.

Reimer, M. S. (1992). Computerized cost analysis for the nursing skills laboratory. *Nurse Educator, 17*(4), 8–11.

Roberts, J., While, A., & Fitzpatrick, J. (1992). Simulation: Current status in nurse education. *Nurse Education Today, 12,* 409–415.

Ullmer, E., & Weisberg, M. (1996). *Computer-based technology in the health sciences: The Learning Center for Interactive Technology.* Bethesda, MD: National Library of Medicine.

The "Resource References" in Chapters 4, 5, and 7, and the "Cataloging and Processing Aids" section in Chapter 6 contain additional references on media, interactive multimedia, CD-ROM, and electronic resources.

APPENDIX A
SELECTED ORGANIZATIONS PROVIDING NURSING MULTIMEDIA RESOURCES

Emerging Technology Consultants
2819 Hamline Avenue, North
St. Paul, MN 55113
Phone: 612-639-3973
Fax: 612-639-0110
E-mail: rpollak@emergingtechnology
   .com
http://www.emergingtechnology.com

FITNE Inc.
5 Depot Street
Athens, OH 45701
Phone: 800-337-4107
Fax: 614-592-2650
http://www.fitne.ev.net

Gale Research, Inc.
835 Penobscot Building
645 Griswold Street
Detroit, MI 48226-4094
Phone: 800-877-4253
Fax: 800-414-5043
E-mail: galeord@gale.com
http://www.gale.com/gale.html

International Communications
   Industries Association
11242 Waples Mill Road
Fairfax, VA 22030
Phone: 703-273-7200
Fax: 703-278-8082
E-mail: icia@icia.org
http://www.icia.org

Lippincott-Raven Publishers
12107 Insurance Way
Haggerstown, MD 21740
Phone: 301-714-2300
Fax: 301-714-2398
http://www.lrpub.com

National Library of Medicine
8600 Rockville Pike
Bethesda, MD 20894
Phone: 800-272-4787
E-mail: publicinfo@nlm.nih.gov
http://www.nlm.nih.gov

Stewart Publishing
4706 Autumn Cove Court
Alexandria, VA 22312
Phone: 703-354-8155
Fax: 703-354-2177
E-mail: stewartpub@aol.com
http://www.interactive-healthcare
   .com

University of Michigan Medical
   Center
Learning Resource Center
Ann Arbor, MI
Phone: 313-763-6770
Fax: 313-763-6771
http://www.med.umich.edu/lrc
   /lrchomepage/lrchome.html

APPENDIX B
CLINICAL SIMULATION LABORATORY:
RESOURCES FOR EQUIPMENT/SUPPLY VENDORS

Anatomical Chart Company
8221 Kimball Ave.
Skokie, IL 60076-2956
Phone: 800-621-7500
Fax: 847-674-0211 or 847-679-9155

Armstrong Medical Industries Inc.
P.O. Box 700
Lincolnshire, IL 60069-0700
Phone: 800-323-4220
Fax: 847-913-0138

Childbirth Graphics, A Division of
    WRS Inc.
P.O. Box 21207
Waco, TX 76702-1207
Phone: 800-299-3366, ext. 287
Fax: 817-751-0221

Gaumard Scientific Company, Inc.
P.O. Box 140098
Coral Gables, FL 33114-0098
Phone: 800-882-6655
Fax: 305-667-6085

General Medical Corporation
8741 Landmark Road
P.O. Box 27452
Richmond, VA 3261-7452
Phone: 800-446-3008

Health Edco, A Division of WRS
    Group, Inc.
P.O. Box 21207
Waco, TX 76702-1207
Phone: 800-229-3366, ext 295
Fax: 817-751-0221

Hill-Rom, A Hillenbrand Industry
1069 State Road, 46 East
Batesville, IN 47006
Phone: 800-638-2546
Fax: 812-934-7191

Hopkins Medical Products
5 Greenwood Place
Baltimore, MD 21208
Phone: 410-484-2036
Fax: 410-484-4036

Laerdale Medical Corporation
167 Myers Comers Road
Wappingers Falls, NY 12590
Phone: 800-431-1055
Fax: 800-227-1143

Medical Plastics Laboratory, Inc.
P.O. Box 38
226 F.M. 116 SO.
Industrial Air Park
Gatesville, TX 76528-0038
Phone: 800-433-5539
Fax: 817-865-8011

Nasco
901 Janesville Ave.
P.O. Box 901
Fort Atkinson, WI 53538-0901
Phone: 800-558-9595
Fax: 414-563-8296

Ohmeda Inc.
Ohmeda Drive
P.O. Box 7550
Madison, WI 53707-7550
Phone: 800-345-2700
Fax: 608-221-4384

Ophthalmic Development Lab
P.O. Box 613
Iowa City, IA 52244

Stryker Medical Group
6300 Sprinkle Road
Kalamazooo, MI 49001
Phone: 800-327-0770

Wallcor Inc.
7720 Clairemont Mesa Boulevard
San Diego, CA 92111-1533
Phone: 619-565-4366
Fax: 619-571-2067

10

Programs and Services of the National Library of Medicine

Dorothy L. Moore, MS, RN

The mission of the National Library of Medicine (NLM) is to collect, organize, preserve, and disseminate the biomedical literature of the world to health professionals in the United States in order to advance the medical and related sciences and to improve the public health. The NLM has a collection of more than 5 million items, including books, journals, audiovisuals, technical reports, microfilms, manuscripts, and pictorial materials. In addition to serving as a national resource for biomedical information, the NLM provides an array of programs and services for use by health professionals, students in the health sciences, and health science librarians. The Library also produces publications and databases and provides education and training for health professionals, information specialist, and librarians; provides grants and contracts for information type projects; and conducts research in biomedical communications.

The U.S. Congress has mandated that the NLM provide information resources and services to all health professionals in the United States, wherever located. To this end, NLM has created,

The author thanks the following for their assistance with this chapter: Cassandra Allen, Becky Lyon, Dr. Angela Ruffin, Carol Vogel, and Frances Beckwith.

distributed, and provided access to a wide body of biomedical information through its online services, printed publications, and its vast collection in Bethesda, Maryland. Among the NLM's targeted groups of health professionals are the thousands of nurses who provide direct health care services to millions of people each day. It is part of the mission of the Library to educate its users about what is available and how to access the many resources and services of NLM, which will fulfill their specific needs.

This chapter provides an overview of some of the programs and services of the National Library of Medicine. Information about ordering publications; tours; hours of operation; grants; training offered to health professionals, librarians, and information specialists; current outreach projects to health professionals; library programs; factsheets; connections to NLM online services; and links to program-area Web servers is available by telephoning 800-272-4787 or through NLM's home page, HyperDoc (http://www.nlm.nih.gov).

BACKGROUND INFORMATION

In 1836 and during the period of U.S. history when nursing was primarily assumed as a function of religious orders, the small collection of books and journals that was to evolve into the National Library of Medicine (NLM) was known as the Library of the Army Surgeon General's Office. As the library developed and its mission broadened over the decades, it occupied a series of temporary homes. In addition, as its name changed, the library gradually became more of a national medical library than a library strictly for the military (Miles, 1982). The Library of the Army Surgeon General became the Army Medical Library in 1922, which became the Armed Forces Medical Library in 1952 (DeBakey, 1991). When the National Library of Medicine Act of 1956 (PL-84-941) was signed by President Eisenhower, the Armed Forces Medical Library was designated the National Library of Medicine and established as a civilian library under the U.S. Public Health Service to ". . . assist the advancement of medical and related sciences, and to aid the dissemination and exchange of scientific and other information important to the progress of medicine and to the public health" (PL 84-941, Sec. 371). The NLM has the Congressional mandate to:

1. Acquire and preserve books, periodicals, prints, films, recordings, and other library materials pertinent to medicine.

2. Organize materials . . . by appropriate cataloging, indexing, and bibliographical listing.

3. Publish and make available catalogs, indexes, and bibliographies . . . .

4. Make available, through loans, photographic or other copying procedures or otherwise, such materials . . . .

5. Provide reference and research assistance.

6. Engage in such other activities in furtherance of the purpose of this part as [the Secretary] deems appropriate and the Library's resources permit (PL 84-941, Sec. 372).

It was further stated in PL 84-941, Section 375, that ". . . for purposes of this part, the terms 'medicine' and 'medical' shall . . . be understood to include preventive and therapeutic medicine, dentistry, pharmacy, hospitalization, nursing, public health, and the fundamental sciences related thereto, and other related fields of study, research, or activity."

In 1962, the National Library of Medicine moved from the Washington Mall building next to the Smithsonian Institution to its new location in Bethesda, Maryland, on the grounds of the National Institutes of Health (NIH). The NLM became a part of NIH in 1968 (DeBakey, 1991, p. 1252). The Lister Hill Center, a 10-story structure, was built adjacent to the 1962 NLM building in 1980 as a part of the NLM.

Three programs have been implemented at the NLM because of the additional need for the coordination, development, and dissemination of information in specialty subject areas:

1. In response to recommendations made by the President's Science Advisory Committee, the Toxicology

Information Program (TIP) was created at the NLM in 1967 to provide toxicology information and data sources (President's Science Advisory Committee, 1966). Subsequent to the recommendations of the NLM Long-Range Planning Committee and the advice of the Board of Regents (NLM, Long-Range Plan, 1993b), indicating a need for environmental and occupational health information resources, the functions of the TIP were subsumed by the Toxicology and Environmental Health Information Program (TEHIP) in 1994.

2. The National Center for Biotechnology Information (NCBI) was established by PL 100-607 in 1988 as a division of the NLM to develop new information methodologies to assist in the understanding of fundamental molecular and genetic processes that control health and disease.

3. The NLM National Information Center on Health Services Research and Health Care Technology (NICHSR) was created at the NLM by the 1993 NIH Revitalization Act, PL 103-43, Subtitle C, to improve ". . . the collection, storage, analysis, retrieval, and dissemination of information on health services research, clinical practice guidelines, and on health care technology, including the assessment of such technology." The NICHSR works closely with the Agency for Health Care Policy and Research to disseminate the results of health services research with special emphasis on clinical practice guidelines.

NURSING INFORMATION AND THE NLM COLLECTION

Materials for the NLM are collected in more than 45 languages and are selected by NLM librarians or are acquired through approval plans with domestic and foreign book vendors, exchange agreements, and the Library of Congress (LC) overseas acquisitions programs. The NLM Technical Services Division coordinates collection development and the selection, acquisition, and processing of all materials. The NLM collection development and retention policies are coordinated with those of the two other major U.S. national libraries, the Library of Congress (LC) and the National Agricultural Library (NAL). Occasionally, joint supplementary policy statements on collecting in specific subject areas or fields are issued with one or both of these national libraries. The 1993 *Collection Development Manual of the National Library of Medicine* and supplementary collection policy statements are available through the NLM gopher (gopher.nlm.nih .gov), the NLM Web home page (http://www.nlm.nih.gov), and from the NLM Office of Public Information (800-272-4787) or the National Technical Information Service, U.S. Department of Commerce, 5285 Port Royal Road, Springfield, VA 22161; telephone: (703) 487-4650.

Nursing is a core subject in the NLM collection. Even in its earliest period of development as a military library, the Library's collection policies reflected a significant interest in collecting nursing materials. For example, in addition to other historical nursing materials, the NLM has the first American edition, first issue, of Florence Nightingale's *Notes on Nursing*, published in 1859; an audio recording of her voice and an autographed copy of her book *Life or Death in India*. The Library also has a signed manuscript presentation copy of a report by Clara Barton to Surgeon General John Moore. Volume 9 of the 1888 *Index-Catalogue of the Library of the Surgeon General's Office* has several pages and over 100 references on "nurses and nursing," published and acquired prior to 1888.

However, because the NLM is a national Library, and ". . . the intent is to ensure that the [permanent] collection represents the intellectual content and diversity of the world's biomedical literature" (National Library of Medicine, 1993a, p. 2), exhaustive collecting of the scholarly literature in core subjects, which includes nursing, does not necessarily extend to ephemera and all formats of materials of the health professions. Hence, there will always be an ongoing need for nursing and the other health professions to provide for the collection of materials relevant to their profession and especially those of historical value.

The NLM receives more than 22,000 serial titles, including journals, indexing and abstracting tools, government documents, and annual reports. Processing for serial procurement, serial gaps (issues and volumes missing from the collection), check-in, and binding are managed by NLM's computerized Master Serials System. Products produced from this system include tools used by biomedical libraries for identifying and locating serials for inter-library loan such as the SERLINE® (SERials onLINE) database, *The List of Journals Indexed for Online Users,* and the quarterly *Health Sciences Serials* microfiche.

Of the serial titles received by the NLM, approximately 3,700 are indexed in MEDLINE® (MEDlars onLine), NLM's most widely used database. Indexing involves analyzing the contents of documents and assigning descriptive headings from NLM's controlled vocabulary, Medical Subject Headings (MeSH®), which has more than 17,000 terms. These assigned subject headings are used by online searchers to retrieve references or citations to items in the NLM databases. Some additional serial titles in the NLM collection are indexed by health science organizations for databases that are developed in collaboration with the NLM, which are also included in NLM's computerized Medical Literature Analysis and Retrieval System (MEDLARS®).

Shortly after the development of MEDLARS, the NLM began a cooperative venture in 1965 with the American Journal of Nursing Company, a subsidiary of the American Nurses Association (ANA), to index the journal literature of nursing (Miles, 1982, p. 376). The citations for articles indexed in nursing journals, in addition to nursing-related subjects for articles in journals indexed for NLM's *Index Medicus,* are identified in MEDLARS and reviewed quarterly in preparation for printing the nursing index. Photocomposed bibliographic records for these citations are then provided to the American Journal of Nursing Company for the *International Nursing Index* (INI).

The first annual cumulation of the INI was published in 1966. Initially, the American Journal of Nursing Company was responsible for selecting the nursing journals that would be indexed for the

INI. This responsibility has since been assumed by the INI Advisory Committee. Citations to articles indexed in nursing journals recommended by consultants serving on NLM's Literature Selection Technical Review Committee are printed in NLM's *Index Medicus*. All of the citations for indexed articles in the INI are included in the MEDLINE database. Not all the nursing serials, including journals, in the NLM collection have been selected for indexing. Along with other nursing serials, these nonindexed nursing journals are included in the SERLINE database.

The National Library of Medicine uses its NLM Classification System for cataloging biomedical materials in its collection, and the LC Classification System is used for cataloging nonbiomedical materials. MeSH® is used for subject cataloging. The NLM Classification System and MeSH are discussed in Chapter 6, Cataloging and Processing.

Materials in the collection of the NLM are available for use by nurses either on-site or through interlibrary loan. The stacks are not open to the public. Information on obtaining material from the NLM on interlibrary loan is discussed in this chapter under "Interlibrary Loan and Document Delivery." Locator, NLM's online catalog, provides Internet access to books, journals, and audiovisuals in the collection. In accessing Locator, use VT-100 emulation and Telnet to locator.nlm.nih.gov, then log in as *locator*. There is no charge for access or usage.

RESOURCE SHARING

The organizational infrastructure for federally supported resource sharing between the National Library of Medicine and other health science libraries in the United States was established when Congress passed the Medical Library Assistance Act (MLAA) of 1965 (PL 89-291). In addition to other provisions, PL 89-291 authorized the National Library of Medicine to provide grants for training in medical library science, special projects, research and development in medical library science and related fields, improving and expanding basic resources of medical libraries and related scientific communication techniques, and financial support of biomedical scientific publications. Most important, the MLAA also authorized the NLM to establish regional medical libraries, and to provide grants and contracts to a small number of existing public or private nonprofit health science libraries to enable each to serve as the regional medical library (RML) for the geographical area in which it is located. The network of regional medical libraries, later to be known as the Regional Medical Library (RML) Network was a means of facilitating a planned systematic sharing of biomedical information resources and services among health sciences libraries. Over the years, the number of regions and regional medical libraries have been as many as 11 and as few as 7.

National Network of Libraries of Medicine™ (NN/LM™)

Despite the resources and services provided to health professionals by the Regional Medical Libraries, it became apparent that there were many health professionals who were not affiliated with health sciences libraries and who still did not have ready and timely access to needed biomedical information. Consequently, in 1987, the U.S. Congress encouraged the NLM ". . . to develop an active outreach program aimed at . . . [the] transfer of the latest scientific findings to all health professionals including psychologists, nurse midwives, and nurse practitioners in rural communities and other areas . . ." (U.S. Congress, Senate, 1987, p. 138).

The National Library of Medicine Act was amended in December of 1987 to require the Library to ". . . publicize the availability of [its] products and services . . ." (U.S. Congress, Joint Resolution, 1987, Sec. 215). Additional funds were provided for outreach. In response to this charge, the NLM Board of Regents convened a Planning Panel on Outreach for the purpose of formulating a plan to guide the library's outreach efforts. The Board of Regents sought a plan that would address the need to increase the awareness of prospective users; suggest strategies for removing obstacles to access; and propose mechanisms to ensure maximum relevance of the Library's diverse array of information products and services. Emphasis would be on access by health professionals in rural areas and inner cities without easy direct access. In 1991, the RML Network was renamed the National Network of Libraries of Medicine (NN/LM). At the same time that the name of the network changed, the network was reconfigured to add an eighth region. Each region has a designated RML. The current designated regions, Regional Medical Libraries and areas served are in Appendix A. The mission of the NN/LM is to provide U.S. health professionals access to NLM biomedical information resources and services. The National Library of Medicine coordinates the NN/LM, which is made up of a nationwide network of more than 4,500 member health science libraries and information centers.

The goals of the NN/LM are to (a) promote an awareness of and access to biomedical information resources for health professionals; (b) develop and improve the biomedical information resources in the regions and support the sharing of these resources within the regions and throughout the United States; and (c) encourage, develop, and support Internet connectivity and inclusion of member libraries and health professionals in the developing National Information Infrastructure (NII). All members of the NN/LM contribute to the achievement of the goals of the network.

Network Membership. Membership in the network is voluntary and self-electing. Applications for membership may be obtained from any of the Regional Medical Libraries or by calling 800 338-7657. Any organization, information center, or library qualifies for membership that has a collection of health sciences materials—for example, books, journals, or audiovisuals—from which it provides one or more of the following information services: interlibrary loan, reference services, or bibliographic searches (manual or computer).

In joining the NN/LM, an organization must designate one employee as a contact for network information and communication. In addition, an organization must agree to be listed in any regional directory produced in its geographic region and in the national registry of network members, and provide basic information about materials and services and other necessary information to

313

the RML every two years for updating the regional directory and national registry of network members.

Categories of Members. The NN/LM is made up of (1) eight Regional Medical Libraries (RMLs), (2) more than 4,400 organizations designated as Primary Access Libraries (PALs), and (3) approximately 140 Resource Libraries (RLs). The NLM administers the NN/LM and serves as backup for the resources of other health science organizations in the network. Many nursing school libraries and health sciences libraries with nursing programs are members of the NN/LM.

Regional Medical Libraries. A library becomes a Regional Medical Library by being awarded a contract by the NLM. These contracts are five-year competitive bid contracts. Regional Medical Libraries must have resources of sufficient depth and scope to supplement the services of other medical libraries within the region served.

The primary responsibilities of Regional Medical Libraries are to:

1. Coordinate and provide health sciences information in their regions.

2. Establish formal agreements with resource or other libraries in its region to provide basic information services to unaffiliated health professionals without charge or on a cost-recovery or fee-for-service basis, and to maintain a directory of libraries providing such information services in the region.

3. Advertise the availability of services available to health professionals through presentations, exhibits, or articles in professional journals, newspapers, and newsletters or other media.

4. Provide interlibrary loans and document delivery to health professionals in conformance with the NN/LM Interlibrary Loan Plan.

5. Conduct targeted outreach programs for unaffiliated, rural, and minority health professionals.

6. Promote the use of Grateful Med® and the National Information Infrastructure (NII) for accessing health science information.

In addition, Regional Medical Libraries conduct research and special projects relating to the dissemination of information, provide consultation and training to librarians and health professionals, and maintain information on local and regional libraries holdings, and submit the information to NLM. RMLs may also provide some funding to other institutions in their regions for outreach projects.

Resource Libraries. A network member may become a Resource Library by being selected by a Regional Medical Library if it meets other specific criteria in addition to the basic qualifications for NN/LM membership. Resource libraries agree to:

1. Participate in regional outreach programs for health professionals, and especially for unaffiliated, rural, minority or inner-city health professionals.

2. Meet network performance standards for interlibrary loan fill rate and throughput time, including fully participating in DOCLINE®, NLM's interlibrary loan and referral system, by sharing health science collection materials and staff expertise.

3. Provide unaffiliated health professionals with access to information services at a reasonable cost.

4. Participate in resource sharing programs in the region.

5. Contribute information on their serial holdings data for inclusion in SERHOLD®, NLM's database, which contains information on the holdings of over 3,000 health science libraries in the United States and Canada.

Primary Access Libraries. The PALs are health science libraries in small local institutions, usually hospitals, that have modest collections and provide services to a clearly defined group of health professionals. PALs need only meet the basic requirements for membership in the NN/LM.

Interlibrary Loan and Document Delivery

The NLM Interlibrary Loan Policy. Much of the book material in the general and historical collections of the NLM is available for interlibrary loan. Journals do not circulate, but NLM provides photocopies of journal articles or scanned images via the Internet for a fee. Some of the historical and brittle monographs and serials in the NLM collection have been microfilmed as a part of the NLM preservation program, and facsimile copies are available for loan or sale. In addition to routine interlibrary loans, NLM will respond to interlibrary loan requests for clinical emergencies within two hours. The NLM does not lend directly to individuals. Following the interlibrary loan policies of the NN/LM, NLM fills requests for materials not held by other libraries. The provisions of the National Interlibrary Loan Code of the American Library Association (ALA) are applicable to all NLM loan requests. Libraries may submit loan requests to the NLM by DOCLINE, ALA or IFLA (International Federation of Library Associations) Interlibrary Loan Request Forms, Internet, or telefacsimile. In addition, the applicable statement of conformance to either the U.S. Copyright Act of 1976 (CCL) or Copyright Guidelines (CCG) must be included with all requests for material to be photocopied. Audiovisual loan requests must include the CCL statement.

Interlibrary Loan and Document Delivery at the Organizational Level. Health sciences organizations planning for interlibrary loan services should obtain a copy of the interlibrary loan policies governing their region from the RML that provides services to their geographical region. In addition, the most recent copies of NLM factsheets should be obtained for general

316

information on the interlibrary loan policies of the NLM, National Network of Libraries of Medicine, National Network of Libraries of Medicine Membership program, access to audiovisuals, online services policy statement, NLM policy on database pricing, SERHOLD, DOCLINE, HyperDoc, Internet connection grants, NLM Internet accessible resources, fixed-fee access, and databases and databanks. Copies of factsheets on these topics are available from NLM's Web page (http://www/nlm.nih.gov) or the Public Information Office (800-272-4787).

Interlibrary Loan and the Individual Nurse. Nurses affiliated with a health sciences library may request photocopies of journal articles and loans of books and audiovisuals through their libraries. Unaffiliated nurses should contact the RML in their region to identify libraries that may provide services to them. See Appendix A for a list of the RMLs. A library provided by the RML should then be contacted to ensure that service is available, and under what conditions.

Nurses using Grateful Med to do their own literature searches may request interlibrary loan from a remote site (e.g., home, office, or clinical area) by using Loansome Doc™, the document-ordering feature of Grateful Med. Grateful Med is a user-friendly microcomputer-based program designed to enable health professionals to search the NLM's MEDLARS databases. Available for the IBM or compatible personal computers (PC) or Apple Macintosh, Grateful Med is easily installed and comes with a tutorial. After completing a search of an NLM database using Grateful Med, the searcher selects references to be ordered from the list of bibliographic citations retrieved from the online search. These references are then ordered electronically using Loansome Doc. Grateful Med searchers should prearrange for services from a member library of the NN/LM that uses DOCLINE prior to using Loansome Doc to request documents. Documents are usually provided for a fee as established by the participating library.

In planning for interlibrary loan, both the affiliated and unaffiliated nurse should especially consider obtaining copies of some of the NLM factsheets previously mentioned in addition to the factsheets on Grateful Med and Loansome Doc.

317

Grateful Med software may be ordered from the U.S. Department of Commerce, National Technical Information Service (NTIS), 5285 Port Royal Road, Springfield, VA 22161. If payment is by credit card, NTIS deposit account, or purchase order, Grateful Med may be ordered from NTIS by telephone, 800-423-9255.

Sharing Resources among Health Science Organizations. Health science libraries, as well as libraries in schools of nursing, have routinely participated in both formal and informal resource-sharing arrangements for cataloging and interlibrary lending prior to the passage of the Medical Library Assistance Act (MLAA) in 1956. Interlibrary loan and document delivery are the major resource-sharing activities among libraries in the NN/LM. To facilitate these processes, each of the eight Regional Medical Libraries have established lending procedures and union lists for their regions. The provisions of the National Interlibrary Loan Code of the American Library Association are applicable in the NN/LM.

To expedite timely access to biomedical information by health professionals, the NLM has developed a number of databases and systems for rapid processing of interlibrary loan requests among health science libraries: DOCLINE, the interlibrary loan request routing and referral system; DOCUSER (DOCument delivery USER), a database that contains the directory, interlibrary loan, and network information on libraries participating in DOCLINE; and SERHOLD®, a database containing the serial holdings of over 3,000 libraries in the United States and in selected Canadian libraries. SERHOLD data provides the basis for the routing of interlibrary loan requests to libraries that have reported owning the requested title.

DOCLINE became operational among the Regional Medical Libraries in 1985. It links to the holdings of approximately 3,000 health science libraries in the United States and Canada in the SERHOLD database. There are currently over 2,800 DOCLINE participants. A health science library, information center, or organization does not have to be a member of the NN/LM in order to be a DOCLINE participant. There is no charge for the use of DOCLINE.

Regional Medical Libraries distribute DOCLINE application packets. Completed applications and interlibrary loan routing tables created by DOCLINE applicants are reviewed by the RMLs prior to being forwarded to the NLM. The NLM assigns DOCLINE codes and unique library identification (LIBID) numbers to institutions, and new DOCLINE users are given a DOCLINE user manual. Manual updates are routinely provided to DOCLINE participants when the system is modified.

When a library or health science organization applies for DOCLINE participation, part of the process is preparation of a routing table indicating the potential lending libraries to which interlibrary loans should be sent. Upon inputting an interlibrary loan request into DOCLINE, routing of the request is based on the established local routing tables provided by the applicant, as well as on the holdings data in the SERHOLD database.

For additional information on DOCLINE, please contact: Collection Access Section; National Library of Medicine; 8600 Rockville Pike; Bethesda, MD 20894; 301-496-5511; 800-633-5666; Internet: ill@nlm.nih.gov.

ONLINE SERVICES

Databases and Databanks

The NLM has: factual databases that provide actual data on subjects, in addition to the sources of the data; bibliographic databases that provide references or citations to publications, some of which have abstracts; and referral databases that direct the user to organizations that focus on specific diseases or health-related issues.

Not all the databases made available to health professionals by the NLM are built or developed by the NLM. Many are built or developed in part or in full by other agencies or organizations. Some are developed as collaborative efforts with the NLM or other government or health professional organizations. A list of the NLM databases, databanks, and other selected electronic sources is provided in Appendix B at the end of this chapter.

Dorothy L. Moore

MeSH, the NLM's controlled vocabulary of subject headings, may be used to search most of the databases built by the NLM and some of the databases built in collaboration with the NLM. Many of the databases made available to the public through MEDLARS but built by other organizations, are indexed with their own controlled vocabularies or keyword systems. Recognizing the problems of searching and retrieving information from databases having information indexed with various and numerous controlled vocabularies and subject heading lists, the NLM conducts ongoing research projects to ameliorate this situation. One such project is the development of a Unified Medical Language System® (UMLS®), intended to facilitate retrieval and integration of biomedical information in electronic format from a variety of sources (Humphreys & Lindberg, 1993). The goal of the UMLS is to make it easy for users to link information from patient care record systems, bibliographic and factual databases, and other electronic information systems. Information about biomedical concepts and terms from many controlled vocabularies are contained in the UMLS Metathesaurus, one of the four knowledge sources that comprise the UMLS. Controlled vocabularies in nursing in the UMLS Metathesaurus include the Classification of Nursing Diagnoses, the Home Health Care Classification of Nursing Diagnoses and Interventions, the Nursing Interventions Classification, and the Omaha System: Applications for Community Health Nursing.

Nurses search the NLM databases through libraries or organizations that are members of the NN/LM or by using Grateful Med to do their own database searching. In addition, some of the NLM databases are available through commercial vendors or on CD-ROM. Various libraries and health sciences organizations also have subsets of the MEDLINE database. To access NLM's databases and databanks online, a searcher needs a microcomputer equipped with a modem or access to the Internet. A MEDLARS user code and a password are also required.

MEDLARS User ID Codes/Passwords. There are no subscription fees or minimum charges associated with the MEDLARS user ID codes. The searcher must however, pay for connect time,

320

the use of computer resources, and the amount of data retrieved for most of the databases.

The NLM offers the following types of MEDLARS user ID codes:

- Regular individual ID codes for health professionals. This code comes with credit introductory practice time.

- Individual student ID codes for college or university students, residents, fellows, or interns. These codes are billed at approximately 50 percent of online charges, except for online prints, automatic SDIs, and OFFSEARCHes, which are billed at the regular rates. No introductory credit practice time is offered. These codes are automatically converted to regular charges after two years. SDIs are searches of the most current month of MEDLINE for the same topic each month. OFFSEARCHes are search strategies submitted during online connect time, stored in the computer, and then processed during nonpeak hours.

- Institutional student ID codes for high school, college or university students, residents, fellows, or interns. These codes may also be assigned to societies that provide online instruction.

Database Pricing Policy. The National Library of Medicine Act of 1956 (PL 84-941) empowers the Secretary of Health and Human Services, with the advice of the NLM Board of Regents, to set policies for the pricing of NLM products and services. One of the philosophical principles underlying the pricing of NLM products and services is that the costs of gaining access to these products and services should be at the lowest feasible price and be shared equally by the biomedical community to the degree possible. The pricing of NLM databases and databanks is reviewed annually. Pricing is computed by connect time, use of computer resources, and the amount of data retrieved or by a fixed or flat rate.

321

An institution may have unlimited Internet access under a fixed-fee arrangement to all NLM nonroyalty databases such as MEDLINE, HealthSTAR, BIOETHICSLINE®, and so on. Royalty fees are charged for the use of CHEMLINE®, TOXLIT®, and TOXLIT65. The annual agreement charge is determined by the size of the user group, the number of user codes required, and previous use of NLM databases from all sources. The fixed fee covers unlimited simultaneous use at multisites by librarians or end users, which may include office, home, or clinical units. Searching may be in command mode (i.e., while using computer command language searching), or by using any or all versions of Grateful Med (DOS, Mac, or Internet GM). The price does not include charges for SDIs and offline prints, which are billed at the regular rates. The fixed-fee agreement offers nursing organizations an opportunity to search the NLM databases at a considerably reduced cost.

A flat-rate agreement provides unlimited Internet access to all NLM nonroyalty databases by individual members of an association that have such an agreement with the NLM. This arrangement provides the opportunity for nursing organizations to provide database searching as a membership benefit.

Using a microcomputer equipped with a modem, one may order Grateful Med and/or obtain a MEDLARS user code and password by Telnet to the Grateful Med Bulletin Board, 800-525-5756. MEDLARS user codes are also assigned through the Internet Grateful Med (IGM) self-registration system (http://igm.nlm .nih.gov). Application packets for online services, which contain application forms for ID codes, setting up fixed-fee and billing accounts, information on billing charges, and NLM online training, are distributed by the NLM MEDLARS Management Section (contact information is given in the next subsection). All MEDLARS user ID codes and assigned passwords are under the administration of the MEDLARS Management Section. Factsheets are available on "NLM Policy on Database Pricing," "NLM Online Charges," and "Fixed-Fee Access."

Online Search Training. In addition to using the self-instructional tutorial included with each copy of Grateful Med, nurses may obtain Grateful Med training through the NN/LM, command language training in classes at the NLM or in the regions, or self-instructional microcomputer-based (IBM or compatible) training. More specific information on online training for searching the NLM databases is available from a Regional Medical Library (800-338-7657) or the NLM MEDLARS Management Section (800-638-8480; e-mail: mms@nlm.nih.gov; TELNET: medlars.nlm.nih.gov).

GRANTS

The NLM Extramural Programs Division provides a range of grants for projects relating to the development, management, and dissemination of biomedical information and technology. The types of grants available for health sciences libraries include resource grants for information access or information systems, Internet connection grants, and Integrated Advanced Information Management Systems (IAIMS). In addition, grants are available to health professionals and librarians for research, publications, and training. Additional information on NLM grants may be obtained by calling 800-272-4787 or via the NLM Web site, http://www.nlm.nih.gov.

NLM INTERNATIONAL MEDLARS CENTERS

Through its international program, the NLM is collaborating and cooperating with public institutions in other countries to make biomedical information available to health professionals in foreign countries. Institutions serving as NLM International MEDLARS Centers have bilateral agreements with the NLM. International MEDLARS Centers provide MEDLARS search services, document delivery, user search assistance, and other information services to health professionals. The centers are capable of using Grateful Med and have Internet access to the MEDLARS databases. The NLM International MEDLARS Centers are listed in Appendix C.

Dorothy L. Moore

CONCLUSION

The National Library of Medicine provides an array of programs and services as a public service for both affiliated and unaffiliated nurses and for organizations providing information resources for nurses. With the assistance of managers of information resources and services for nurses and members of the NN/LM, nurses can acquire the skills and knowledge necessary to access and use these resources for application in educational, clinical and administrative settings.

REFERENCES

DeBakey, M. E. (1991). The National Library of Medicine: Evolution of a premier information center. *JAMA, 266,* 1252–1258.

Humphreys, B. L., & Lindberg, D. A. B. (1993). The UMLS project: Making the conceptual connection between users and the information they need. *Bulletin of the Medical Library Association, 81,* 170–177.

Miles, W. D. (1982). *A history of the National Library of Medicine: The nation's treasury of medical knowledge.* Bethesda, MD: National Library of Medicine.

National Library of Medicine. (1993a). *Collection development manual of the National Library of Medicine* (3rd ed.). Bethesda, MD: National Library of Medicine.

National Library of Medicine. (1993b). *Long-range plan; Improving toxicology and environmental health information services; report of the NLM Board of Regents.* Bethesda, MD: National Library of Medicine.

President's Science Advisory Committee. (1966). *Handling of toxicological information.* Washington, DC: The White House.

U.S. Congress. (1987). *Joint Resolution Amending the National Library of Medicine Act, Public Law 100-202, Section 215.*

U.S. Congress, Senate, Committee on Appropriations. (1988). *Departments of Labor, Health and Human Services, and Education and Related Agencies Appropriation Bill, 1988: Report to Accompany H.R. 3058, 100th Cong., 1st sess., 1987, S.Rept. 100-189, p. 138.*

U.S. Congress, Senate, Committee on Appropriations. (1988). *Departments of Labor, Health and Human Services, and Education and Related Agencies Appropriation Bill, 1989: Report to accompany H.R. 4783, 100 Cong., 2nd sess, 1988. S. Rept. 100-399, p. 145.*

SUGGESTED READINGS

Byrnes, M. M. (1989). Preservation of the biomedical literature: An overview. *Bulletin of the Medical Library Association, 77,* 269–275.

Clyman, J. L., Powsner, S. M., Paton, J. A., & Miller, P. L. (1993). Using a network menu and the UMLS Information Sources Map to facilitate access to online reference materials. *Bulletin of the Medical Library Association, 81,* 207–216.

Corn, M., & Johnson, F. E. (1994). Connecting the health sciences community to the Internet: The NLN/NSF grant program. *Bulletin of the Medical Library Association, 82,* 392–395.

Dorsch, J. L., & Landwirth, T. K. (1993). Rural GRATEFUL MED outreach: Project results, impact, and future needs. *Bulletin of the Medical Library Association, 81,* 377–382.

Dugan, R. E., Cheverie, J. F., & Souza, J. L. (1996). The NII: For the public good. In Information Policy, R. E. Dugan & P. Heron (Eds.), *The Journal of Academic Librarianship.*

Martin E. R., & Lanier, D. (1995). Delivering medical information to the desktop: The UIC GRATEFUL-MED-via-the-Internet experience. *Bulletin of the Medical Library Association, 83,* 402–406.

McClure, C. R. (1996). Libraries and federal information policy. In *Information Policy,* edited by R. E. Dugan & P. Hernon. *The Journal of Academic Librarianship, 22,* 214–218.

Schuyler, P. L., & Hole, W. T. (1993). The UMLS Metathesaurus: Representing different views of biomedical concepts. *Bulletin of the Medical Library Association, 81,* 217–222.

Willmering, W. J., Fishel, M. R., & McCutcheon, D. E. (1988). SERHOLD: Evolution of the national biomedical serials holdings database. *Serials Review, 14*(1–2), 7–13.

Zink, S., Illes, J., & Vannier, M. W. (1996). NLM extramural program. Frequently asked questions. *Bulletin of the Medical Library Association, 84,* 165–181.

Dorothy L. Moore

APPENDIX A
REGIONS, REGIONAL MEDICAL LIBRARIES,
AND AREAS SERVED

1. Middle Atlantic Region
The New York Academy of Medicine
1216 Fifth Avenue
New York, NY 10029
Phone: 212-822-7300
Fax: 212-534-7042
URL: http://www.nnlm.nlm.nih.gov/mar
States served: DE, NJ, NY, PA
National Online Center for All Regions

2. Southeastern/Atlantic Region
University of Maryland at Baltimore
Health Sciences Library
111 South Greene Street
Baltimore, MD 21201-1583
Phone: 410-706-2855
Fax: 410-706-0099
URL: http://www.nnlm.nlm.nih.gov/sar
States served: AL, FL, GA, MD, MS, NC, SC, TN, VA, WV, the District of
    Columbia, Puerto Rico, and the U.S. Virgin Islands

3. Greater Midwest Region
University of Illinois at Chicago
Library of the Health Sciences (M/C 763)
1750 W. Polk Street
Chicago, IL 60612-7223
Phone: 312-996-2464
Fax: 312-996-2226
URL: http://www.nnlm.nlm.nih.gov/gmr
States served: IA, IL, IN, KY, MI, MN, ND, OH, SD, WI

4. Midcontinental Region
University of Nebraska Medical Center
Leon S. McGoogan Library of Medicine
600 South 42nd Street
Omaha, NE 68198-6706
Phone: 402-559-4326
Fax: 402-559-5482
URL: http://www.nnlm.nlm.nih.gov/mr
States served: CO, KS, MO, NE, UT, WY

5. South Central Region
Houston Academy of Medicine
Texas Medical Center Library
1133 M.D. Anderson Boulevard
Houston, TX 77030-2809
Phone: 713-790-7053
Fax: 713-790-7030
URL: http://www.nnlm.nlm.nih.gov/scr
States served: AR, LA, NM, OK, TX

6. Pacific Northwest Region
University of Washington
Health Sciences Library and Information Center
P.O. Box 357155
Seattle, WA 98195-7155
Phone: 206-543-8262
Fax: 206-543-2469
URL: http://www.nnlm.nlm.nih.gov/pnr
States served: AK, ID, MT, OR, WA

7. Pacific Southwest Region
University of California, Los Angeles
Louise M. Darling Biomedical Library
12-077 Center for Health Sciences
P.O. Box 951798
Los Angeles, CA 90095-1798
Phone: 301-825-1200
Fax: 301-825-5389
URL: http://www.nnlm.nlm.nih.gov/psr
States served: AZ, CA, HI, NV, and
    US Territories in the Pacific Basin

8. New England Region
University of Connecticut Health Center
Lyman Maynard Stowe Library
263 Farmington Avenue
Farmington, CT 06030-5370
Phone: 860-679-4500
Fax: 860-679-1305
URL: http://www.nnlm.nlm.nih.gov/ner
States served: CT, MA, ME, NH, RI, VT

Dorothy L. Moore

APPENDIX B
NLM DATABASES, DATABANKS, AND
SELECTED OTHER ELECTRONIC RESOURCES

AIDSDRUGS. AIDSDRUGS is a dictionary file of over 240 chemical and biological agents currently being evaluated in AIDS clinical trials, which are covered in the companion AIDSTRIALS database. Each record represents a single substance and provides information such as CAS Registry Numbers, standard chemical names, synonyms, trade names, protocol ID numbers, pharmacological action, adverse reactions and contraindications, physical/chemical properties, and manufacturers' names. Agents tested in closed or completed trials are also included. Relevant articles are also included. English language. Updated monthly. No fee charged for access.

AIDSLINE® (AIDS information onLINE). AIDSLINE includes bibliographic citations to over 124,000 journal articles, government reports, letters, technical reports, meeting abstracts/papers, monographs, special publications, theses, books, and audiovisuals on Acquired Immunodeficiency Syndrome (AIDS) and related topics. Articles cover research, clinical aspects, and health policy issues. Citations are derived from the MEDLINE, CANCERLIT, HealthSTAR, CATLINE, AVLINE, and BIOETHICSLINE files; meeting abstracts from newsletters and special AIDS-related meetings, symposia and conferences; and abstracts and citations from newsletters and special AIDS journals. All languages; publications from 1980 to the present; updated weekly. No fee charged for access.

AIDSTRIALS (AIDS clinical TRIALS). AIDSTRIALS contains over 700 records of clinical trials of substances being tested for use against AIDS, HIV infection, and AIDS-related opportunistic diseases. Each record covers a single trial, and provides information such as title and purpose of the trial, diseases studied, patient eligibility criteria, contact persons, agents being tested, and trial locations. The National Institute of Allergy and Infectious Diseases (NIAID) provides the information about the trials, sponsored by the National Institutes of Health (NIH); information about privately sponsored trials is provided by the Food and Drug Administration (FDA). AIDSTRIALS is a part of the AIDS Clinical Trials Information Service (ACTIS), which is a U.S. Public Health Service project sponsored by the NLM, FDA,

328

NIAID, and the Centers for Disease Control (CDC). Updated bi-weekly. No fee charged for access.

AVLINE® (AudioVisuals on LINE). AVLINE contains bibliographic citations to over 29,000 primarily English-language biomedical audiovisual materials and computer software cataloged by the NLM since 1975, plus clinical educational materials and audiovisual/computer software serials. Selected citations include abstracts. Procurement information available at the time of cataloging is included. Updated weekly. No fee charged for access.

BIOETHICSLINE® (BIOETHICS onLINE). BIOETHICSLINE contains over 48,000 bibliographic citations to journal articles, monographs, analytics (chapters in monographs), newspaper articles, court decisions, bills, laws, audiovisual materials, and unpublished documents on ethics and related public policy issues in health care and biomedical research. Topics include euthanasia and other end-of-life issues, organ donation and transplantation, allocation of health care resources, patients' rights, professional ethics, new reproductive technologies, genetic intervention, abortion, behavior control and other mental health issues, AIDS, human experimentation, and animal experimentation. Citations are derived from the literature of law, religion, the social sciences, philosophy, and the popular media, as well as the health sciences. The file is produced by the Bioethics Information Retrieval Project of the Kennedy Institute of Ethics at Georgetown University. Updated bi-monthly. English-language citations from 1973 to present.

CANCERLIT® (CANCER LITerature) CANCERLIT contains over 1,200,000 bibliographic records of journal articles, government reports, technical reports, meeting abstracts and papers, monographs, letters, and theses, some published as early as 1963 on major cancer topics; it is comprehensive and international since 1976. Since June 1983, most journal literature has been derived from MEDLINE. Records added since January 1980 have been indexed using MeSH, the NLM controlled vocabulary. CANCERLIT is produced by the National Cancer Institute (NCI) in cooperation with the NLM. Updated monthly.

CCRIS (Chemical Carcinogenesis Research Information System). CCRIS is a factual databank of over 7,000 records on carcinogenicity, tumor promotion, tumor inhibition, and mutagenicity test

results derived from the scanning of primary journals, current awareness tools, National Cancer Institute (NCI) technical reports, review
articles, and International Agency for Research on Cancer monographs
published since 1976. Test results have been reviewed by experts in carcinogenesis, and are organized by chemical record . CCRIS is sponsored
by the NCI. Updated monthly.

CATLINE® (CATalog onLINE).   CATLINE contains over 760,000
bibliographic records of primarily monographs, some serials, monograph-
ics series, and manuscripts. It includes records in all languages, and virtually all of the cataloged titles in the NLM collection, from the fifteenth
century to the present. CATLINE provides access to NLM's authoritative bibliographic data, and is a useful source of information for providing reference services, for ordering printed material, and for verifying
interlibrary loan requests. Updated weekly. No fee charged for access.

ChemID® (CHEMical IDentification).   ChemID is a dictionary
file containing records on over 287,000 compounds of biomedical and
regulatory interest. Records include CAS Registry Numbers and other
identifying numbers, molecular formulae, generic names, trivial names;
and other synonyms, MeSH headings, and file locators, which lead
users to other files on the ELHILL and TOXNET systems. The
SUPERLIST also provides names and other data used to describe
chemicals on over 30 key federal and state regulatory lists. Updated
quarterly.

CHEMLINE® (CHEMical dictionary onLINE).   CHEMLINE is
a dictionary file containing records on over 1,400,000 chemical substances found in the NLM databases, the Toxic Substances Control Act
Inventory of the Environmental Protection Agency, the European Inventory of Existing Commercial Chemical Substances (EINECS), and
the Domestic Substances List of Canada. Each record provides detailed
information on the chemical substance's nomenclature, synonyms,
and CAS Registry Numbers. NLM file locators direct the user to
MEDLARS files, which contain more information about the designated
substances. CHEMLINE is produced by NLM's Specialized Information Services with contract support from Chemical Abstracts Service
(CAS). Updated bimonthly. Royalty charges apply.

DART® (Developmental and Reproductive Toxicology).   DART
contains over 28,000 bibliographic citations on biological, chemical,

and physical agents that may cause birth defects. Records include bibliographic citations, abstracts (when available), chemical names, and CAS Registry Numbers. International in coverage, with publications dating from 1989 to the present; it continues the ETICBACK database. DART is produced by the Environmental Protection Agency (EPA), the National Institute of Environmental Health Sciences (NIEHS), and the National Center for Toxicological Research (NCTR) in cooperation with the NLM. Updated periodically.

DENTALPROJ. DENTALPROJ is a factual and referral database that provides information on over 850 ongoing dental research projects, including project summaries, title, name of principal investigator, performing institution, sponsoring organization, and a brief abstract of the project. This database is produced by the National Institute of Dental Research (NIDR) in cooperation with the NLM. Updated semiannually.

DIRLINE® (Directory of Information Resources onLINE). DIRLINE contains over 17,000 records on resource centers, including health-related organizations, government agencies, information centers, professional societies, voluntary associations, support groups, academic and research institutions, and research facilities and resources willing to respond to public inquiries in their specialty areas. Records include addresses, resource names, telephone numbers, and descriptions of services, publications, and holdings. Updated quarterly.

DOCUSER® (DOCument delivery USER). DOCUSER is a file of over 14,000 health-related libraries and other information-related organizations located in the United States and about 1,700 foreign libraries, which use NLM's interlibrary loan services or are a part of the National Network of Libraries of Medicine. For each organization, descriptive and administrative information includes institutional identification, interlibrary loan policy data, participation in the National Network of Libraries of Medicine, and SERHOLD reporting data. Updated monthly.

EMIC and EMICBACK (Environmental Mutagen Information Center BACKfile). EMICBACK contains over 88,000 bibliographic citations to chemical, biological, and physical agents that have been tested for genotoxic activity. The records include full bibliographic references, keywords, chemical names, and CAS Registry Numbers. The file is produced by the Oak Ridge National Laboratory in cooperation with the NLM and funded by the EPA and the NIEHS. International in coverage with publications from 1950–1995; a small number of older citations are found in EMICBACK. Recent citations (1992 and later) are in the EMIC database.

ENTREZ Molecular Sequence Database System. The Entrez sequence databases presents an integrated view of DNA and protein sequence data, 3D structure data, and associated MEDLINE entries; includes protein and nucleotide sequence data from GenBank, DDBJ, PIR-International, PRF, EMBL, Swiss-Prot, and PDB; also includes a molecular biology MEDLINE subset. For information on access, contact the NLM National Center for Biotechnology Information (NCBI) by e-mail: net-info@ncbi.nlm.nih.gov.

ETICBACK (Environmental Teratology Information Center BACKfile). ETICBACK contains about 50,000 bibliographic records on agents that may cause birth defects. The records include bibliographic citations, ETIC keywords, chemical names, and CAS Registry Numbers. ETICBACK was funded by the agency for Toxic Substances and Disease Registry (ATSDR), the EPA, and the NIEHS. International in coverage with publications dating from 1950–1989, and a small number of older citations. Recent citations (1989 and later) are included in the DART (Developmental and Reproductive Toxicology) database.

GENE-TOX (GENetic TOXicology). GENE-TOX, created by the Environmental Protection Agency, contains about 2,900 records on chemicals tested for mutagenicity. Includes peer-reviewed data. No routine schedule for updates.

HealthSTAR™ (Health Services, Technology, Administration, and Research). HealthSTAR contains clinical information emphasizing the evaluation of patient outcomes and the effectiveness of procedures, programs, products, services, and processes and nonclinical information emphasizing the health care administration and planning aspects of health care delivery. It combines the former HEALTH (Health Planning and Administration) and HSTAR (Health Service/ Technology Assessment Research) databases. Bibliographic records are from journal articles, technical and government reports, books and book chapters, and meeting papers and abstracts. These bibliographic records are subsets of MEDLINE (1975 to present) and CATLINE (1985 to present), and are from: (1) records emphasizing health care administration selected and indexed by the American Hospital

Association (AHA); (2) records emphasizing health planning from the National Health Planning Information Center (only in the backfile); and (3) records emphasizing health services research, health care technology assessment, and clinical practice guidelines selected and indexed through NLM National Information Center on Health Services Research and Health Care Technology (NICHSR). This database is produced by the AHA in cooperation with the NLM. The *Hospital and Health Administration Index,* published by the AHA, is produced from this database. Alternate source information that may not be widely available in libraries is provided for technical reports and related material selected by NICHSR staff.

The database is divided into two files based on year of publication: current file, covering 1990 to the present; and a backfile covering 1975 through 1989. It is primarily English language, but international in scope; the current and backfile together contain about 2.5 million records. The database is updated weekly, except for the records from CATLINE, which are added monthly.

HISTLINE® (HISTory of medicine onLINE). HISTLINE contains about 155,000 bibliographic records on the history of health-related professions, sciences, specialties, individuals, institutions, drugs, and diseases of the world and all historic periods. It contains citations to monographs, journal articles, book chapters, and individual chapters in the published proceedings of symposia, congresses, and so on. Virtually all records of secondary historical literature from MEDLINE, CATLINE, and AVLINE are included in HISTLINE. Also included are records that have been indexed by the History of Medicine Division, which are not available from any other MEDLARS database. All languages. Updated weekly; has publications from 1964 to present.

HSDB® (Hazardous Substances Data Bank). HSDB is a factual databank of over 4,500 records, organized by chemical record. Covers hazardous chemicals, toxic effects, environmental fate, and safety and handling of chemicals. The file is enhanced with the data from such related areas as emergency handling procedures, human exposure, detection methods, and regulatory requirements. HSDB contains complete references for all data sources utilized. The file is fully peer-reviewed by the Scientific Review Panel (SRP), a committee of expert toxicologists and other scientists. Data are derived from a core set of standard texts and monographs, government documents, technical reports, and the primary journal literature. Updated continuously.

HSRPROJ (Health Services Research Projects in Progress). HSRPROJ contains about 3,000 records on health services research projects, including health technology assessment and the development and use of clinical practice guidelines from monographs, journal articles, publications from symposia and congresses. Coverage is primarily for the United States, with increasing coverage of international research. It provides project records for research in progress funded by federal and private grants and contracts. Records include project summaries, names of performing and sponsoring agencies, names and addresses of the principal investigator, beginning and ending years of the project, and when available, information about the study design and methodology. Records are indexed with MeSH, and when available, CRISP (Computer Retrieval of Information on Scientific Projects) keywords on records selected from the NIH CRISP information system. Updated quarterly.

HSTAT (Health Services/Technology Assessment Text). HSTAT is an electronic resource that provides access to full-text clinical practice guidelines, quick-reference guides for clinicians, consumer brochures sponsored by the Agency for Health Care Policy and Research (AHCPR); technology assessment reports, NIH consensus research protocols, and HIV/AID Treatment Information Service resources documents; U.S. Public Health Service (PHS) *Preventive Services Task Force Guide to Clinical Preventive Services;* and the Substance Abuse and Mental Health Services Administration, Center for Substance Abuse Treatment (SAMHSA/CSAT) treatment improvement protocols. Access: http://text.nlm.nih.gov/; also accessible with software clients such as Gopher, through Telnet and FTP.

Images from the History of Medicine (IHM). IHM contains about 60,000 historical images from NLM's collection of caricatures, photographs, fine prints, portraits, ephemera, and illustrations drawn from books and journals in the NLM collection. Access: http://www.nlm.nih.gov.

IRIS (Integrated Risk Information System). IRIS is a factual database containing over 660 records on potentially toxic chemicals and chemical-specific EPA health risk and regulatory information prepared by the Environmental Protection Agency. The NLM version of the file includes oral reference doses and inhalation reference concentrations for noncarcinogens, and data such as slope factors and unit risks for carcinogens. Toxic risk data undergo a high level of scientific review. Updated monthly.

MEDLINE® (MEDlars onLINE). MEDLINE contains over 8.5 million bibliographic citations to articles from more than 3,700 international biomedical journals, dating from 1966 to the present, in all languages. Recent references are contained in the current file (MEDLINE); segmented MEDLINE Backfiles (MED90, MED85, MED80, MED75, and MED66) contain older material. Updated daily, except in November and December. The citations for each monthly update are also searchable in a separate file called SDILINE® (Selective Dissemination of information onLINE), covering the fields of medicine, nursing, dentistry, veterinary medicine, and the preclinical sciences. MEDLINE contains all citations published in *Index Medicus®*, and corresponds in part to the *International Nursing Index* and the *Index to Dental Literature*. Citations include the English abstract when published with the article (approximately 75 percent of the current file).

MeSH VOCABULARY FILE®. The MeSH Vocabulary File is an online dictionary or thesaurus of current biomedical subject headings, subheadings, and supplementary chemical terms used in indexing and searching several MEDLARS databases. Updated annually, it contains about 18,000 medical subject headings and over 87,000 supplementary chemical records.

PDQ® (Physician Data Query). PDQ is a factual and referral database containing current information on cancer treatment and clinical trials in the United States, Canada, and Western Europe. It provides detailed information on the prognosis, staging, and treatment of all major tumor types, screening for common cancers, supportive care for common problems encountered in cancer patients, summaries of open and closed clinical trials, directories of physicians and organizations providing cancer care and information on investigational cancer drugs. Updated monthly.

POPLINE® (POPulation information on LINE). POPLINE contains over 230,000 primarily English-language bibliographic citations to journal articles, monographs, technical reports, and unpublished works on family planning technology and programs, fertility, population law and policy, and primary health care, including maternal/child health in developing countries. Produced by the Population Information

335

Dorothy L. Moore

Program at the Johns Hopkins School of Public Health. The database is funded primarily by the United States Agency of International Development. Updated monthly.

RTECS® (Registry of Toxic Effects of Chemical Substances). This factual databank contains about 132,000 records on potentially toxic chemicals focusing on the acute and chronic effects of potentially toxic chemicals; data on skin/eye irritation, carcinogenicity, mutagenicity, and reproductive consequences are included. Selected federal regulatory requirements and exposure levels are also presented. References are available for all data; toxicology and carcinogenic reviews, when available, are cited. RTECS is built and maintained by the National Institute for Occupational Safety and Health (NIOSH). Updated quarterly.

SDILINE® (Selective Dissemination of Information onLINE). SDILINE contains bibliographic citations in all languages from the most recent complete month in MEDLINE, including all citations in the forthcoming printed edition of the monthly *Index Medicus*. Updated monthly, with about 31,000 new citations to journal articles from approximately 3,700 biomedical journals published in the United States and abroad.

SERLINE® (SERials onLINE). SERLINE contains bibliographic citations to about 87,000 biomedical serial titles in all languages published from 1665 to the present. It lists bibliographic records for all serials cataloged for the NLM collection; titles ordered or being processed for the NLM; and all serial titles indexed for MEDLINE and HealthSTAR, including titles that do not meet NLM scope and coverage requirements; also includes titles held by libraries participating in the NLM National Biomedical Serials Holdings Database (SERHOLD®) and record locator information that identifies the holdings of biomedical libraries within the National Network of Libraries of Medicine.

SPACELINE™. SPACELINE contains about 100,000 bibliographic citations to journal articles; technical reports; books and book chapters; conference proceedings, conference papers, and meeting abstracts; bibliographies; and audiovisuals in all languages on space life sciences; all references in scope from MEDLINE (1966 to the present), CATLINE, and AVLINE, plus thousands of citations from

336

1961 to the present contributed by NASA. The file became available in October 1995. SPACELINE is a cooperative venture of NLM and the National Aeronautics and Space Administration (NASA). Its purpose is to consolidate the growing body of space life sciences research into a single, easily accessible resource.

TOXLINE® (TOXicology information onLINE). TOXLINE and TOXLINE65 together contain over 2 million primarily English-language bibliographic citations to journal articles, monographs, technical reports, theses, letters, and meeting abstracts, papers and reports on toxicological, pharmacological, biochemical, and physiological effects and drugs and other chemicals. Coverage is international. The database has been segmented: pre-1965 to 1980 material is found in TOXLINE65, and 1981-forward citations are found in the TOXLINE file. The database is made up of about 16 secondary sources, which do not require royalty charges based on usage.

TOXLIT® (TOXicology LITerature from special sources). TOXLIT® contains over 2 million primarily English-language bibliographic citations to journal articles, meeting papers, monographs, and patents on toxicological, pharmacological, biochemical, and physiological effects of drugs and other chemicals. International in coverage. The database has been segmented: pre-1965 to 1980 citations are found in TOXLIT65, and 1981-forward citations are found in the TOXLIT file. Citations are derived exclusively from Chemical Abstracts. Royalty charges apply.

TRI (Toxic Chemical Release Inventory) series. The TRI series contains the annual estimated release of toxic chemicals to the environment, amounts transferred to waste sites, and source reduction and recycling data; includes numeric data for industrial submissions reported to EPA for the years 1987, 1988, 1989, 1990, 1991, 1992, 1993, and 1994. A new file is added annually: TRI87 contains over 80,000 records; TRI88 contains over 87,000 records; TRI89 contains over 87,000 records; TRI90 contains about 87,000 records; TRI91 contains about 85,000 records; TRI92 contains over 82,000 records; TRI93 contains over 80,000 records; TRI94 will contain about 80,000 records.

TRI is a series of nonbibliographic files based upon data submitted by industrial facilities around the country to the EPA as mandated by section 313 of the Emergency Planning and Community Right-to-Know

Dorothy L. Moore

Act. TRI records include the names and addresses of industrial facilities releasing toxic chemicals, the amounts released to air, water, land, or by underground injection, and the amounts transferred to waste sites. Files after TRI91 contain source-reduction and recycling data as mandated by the Pollution Prevention Act of 1990. TRI93 contains data on chemicals released by federal facilities, which is supplied on a voluntary basis by some government agencies.

TRIFACTS (Toxic Chemical Release Inventory FACTSheets). TRIFACTS is intended as a companion to the TRI series, and based largely upon the State of New Jersey's Hazardous Substance Factsheets. Designed for a lay audience, these 326 records present scientifically accepted information in nontechnical language, and include health, ecological effects, safety, and handling information for most of the chemicals listed in the TRI (Toxic Chemical Release Inventory) files. No routine schedule for updating.

APPENDIX C
NLM INTERNATIONAL MEDLARS CENTERS

AUSTRALIA
National Library of Australia
Canberra ACT 2603, AUSTRALIA
Phone: 61-6-262-1326
Fax: 61-6-273-1180
E-mail: m.newman@nla.gov.au
URL: http://www.nla.gov.au

CANADA
Canada Institute for Scientific and
Technical Information (CISTI)
National Research Council of
    Canada
Ottawa, Ontario K1A OS2,
    CANADA
Phone: 800-668-1222
Fax: 613-952-8244
E-mail: cisti.medlars@nrc.ca
URL: http://www.cisti.nrc.ca
    /cisti/cisti.html

CHINA
Institute of Medical Information
Chinese Academy of Medical
    Sciences
3, Yabao Road, Choyang District
Beijing 10002, CHINA
Phone: 8610-512-8185
Fax: 8610-512-8176
E-mail: wangrk@bepc2.ihep.ac.cn
URL: http://www.imicams.ac.cn

EGYPT
Academy of Scientific Research and
    Technology
P.O. Box 1522, Attaba 11511
Cairo, EGYPT
Phone: 202-355-7253
Fax: 202-354-7807
E-mail: ab@enstinet.eg.net
URL: http://www.sti.sci.eg

FRANCE
INSERM
101, rue de Tolbiac
75654 Paris Cedex 13, FRANCE
Phone: 33-1-44-23-60-70
Fax: 33-1-44-23-60-99
E-mail: advocat@inserm-dicdoc
   .u-strasbg.fr
URL: http://www-inserm.u-strasbg.fr

GERMANY
Deutsches Institute for Medical
   Documentation and Information
   (DIMDI)
Postfach 420580, D-50899
Koln, GERMANY
Phone: 49-221-472-4252
Fax: 49-221-41-1429
URL: http://www.dimdi.de

HONG KONG
The Chinese University of Hong
   Kong (CUHK)
Prince of Wales Hospital
Li Ping Medical Library
Shantin, N.T., HONG KONG
Phone: 852-2632-2466
Fax: 852-2637-7817
E-mail: medref@cuhk.edu.hk
URL: http://www.lib.cuhk.hk
   /medlib/mdmain.htm

INDIA
National Informatics Center
Planning Commission
A-Block, CGO Complex, Lodi Road
New Delhi 110003, INDIA
Phone: 91-11-436-2359
Fax: 91-11-436-2628
E-mail: root@medlar0.delhi.nic.in

ISRAEL
Hebrew University, Hadassah
   Medical School
Berman National Medical Library
P.O. Box 12272
Jerusalem 91120, ISRAEL
Phone: 972-2-758-795
Fax: 972-2-758-376
E-mail: ester@mdlib.huji.ac.il

ITALY
Ministry of Health
Istituto Superiore di Sanita
Viale Regina Elena 299
00161 Rome, ITALY
Phone: 39-6-499-2280
Fax: 39-6-444-0246
E-mail: dracos@iss.it
URL: http://www.iss.it

JAPAN
Japan Science and Technology
   Corporation (JST)
Information Center for Science and
   Technology
Department of Information
   Resources Management
5-3, Yonbancho,
Chiyoda ku, Tokyo, 102 JAPAN
Phone: 81-3-5214-8407
Fax: 81-3-5214-8470
URL: http://www.jicst.go.jp

KOREA
Medical Library
Seoul National University
College of Medicine
28 Yongon-dong, Chongno-gu
Seoul 110-799, KOREA
Phone: 822-740-8044
Fax: 822-744-0484

KUWAIT
Ministry of Public Health
Kuwait Institute for Medical
   Specialization
P.O. Box 1793 Safat
Code 13018, KUWAIT
Phone: 965-247 2210
Fax: 965-241-0028

Dorothy L. Moore

MEXICO
Centro Nacional de Informacion y
  Documentacion
sobre Salud (CENIDS)
Leibnitz #20, 3er, piso, Colonia
  Anzures
Delegacion Benito Juarez
11590 Mexico D. F., MEXICO
Phone: 525-563-27-82
Fax: 525-598-21-78
E-mail: gladys@cenids.ssa.gob.mx
URL: http://www.ssa.gob.mx/

SOUTH AFRICA
South African Medical Research
  Council
P.O. Box 19070
Tygerberg 7505, SOUTH AFRICA
Phone: 27-21-938-0219
Fax: 27-21-938-0201
E-mail: jalouw@eagle.mrc.ac.za
URL: http://www.mrc.ac.za

SWEDEN
Medical Information Center
Karolinska Institute,
S-171-77 Stockholm, SWEDEN
Phone: 46-8-728-8000
Fax: 46-8-330-0481
E-mail: goran.falkenberg@micforum
  .ki.se
URL: http://www.mic.ki.se

SWITZERLAND
Documentation Service of the Swiss
  Academy of Medical Sciences
  (DOKDI)
Effingerstrasse 40
P.O. Box 5921, 3001 Bern,
  SWITZERLAND
Phone: 41-31-389-92-22
Fax: 41-31-389-92-45
E-mail: dokdi@sams.ch
URL: http://www.sams.ch

UNITED KINGDOM
The British Library
Boston Spa, Wetherby

West Yorkshire LS23 7BQ,
  UNITED KINGDOM
Phone: 44-1-937-546419
Fax: 44-1-937-546458
E-mail: blink-helpdesk@bl.uk
URL: http://portico.bl.uk/sris
  /leadmed.html

PAN AMERICAN HEALTH
  ORGANIZATION (PAHO)
Headquarters, Room 854
525 Twenty-third Street, N. W.
Washington, DC 20037
Phone: 202-861-3212
Fax: 202-223-5971
E-mail: gamboa@nlm.nih.gov
URL: http://www.bireme.br/

BIREME/PAHO
Centro Latino Americano e de
  Caribe
Informcao em Ciencias da Saude
Organizacao Pan-Americana da Saude
Rua Botucatu 862
Vila Clementino, 04023, SP-901
Sao Paulo, BRAZIL
Phone: 55-11-549-2611
Fax: 55-11-571-1919
E-mail: celia@bireme.br
URL: http://www.bireme.br/

INTERGOVERNMENTAL
  ORGANIZATION
Science and Technology Information
  Center
106, Sec. 2, Ho-Ping E. Rd.
Taipei 10636, TAIWAN
Phone: 886-2-737-7690
Fax: 886-2-737-7664
E-mail: sheu@mailsrv.st.stic.gov.tw
URL: http://192.83.171.250

Index

Index

American Association for the History of Nursing (AAHN), 237
American Association of College of Nursing (AACN):
certification programs, 5
Position Statement on Nursing's Agenda for the 21st Century, 8
American Association of Critical-Care Nurses, 17–18
American Association of Industrial Nurses Journal, 19
American College of Physicians, 155
American Journal of Nursing, 19, 145, 155, 166, 170
American Journal of Nursing Company, 19, 225, 310
American Library Association (ALA):
accreditation, 82
American Colleges and Research Libraries, 114–115
continuing education programs, 84
Filing Rules, 115
Intellectual Freedom Manual, 52
Library Bill of Rights, 49–51
National Interlibrary Loan Code, 316, 318
new media resources, 165
promotional materials, 93
Reference and Adult Services Division, 126
standards, 52
American Medical Informatics Association, 84
American National Standards Institute (ANSI), 35
American Nurse Credentialing Center (ANCC), 5–6
American Nurses Association (ANA):
American Journal of Nursing Company, 310
archives, 225
certification and, 5–6
historical perspective, 3
overview of, 16
publications, 110–111, 159–160

American Nursing, a Bibliographical Dictionary, 195
American Society of Information Scientists, 84
American Society of Superintendents of Training Schools for Nurses, 16
American Society of Testing Materials (ASTM), 256
Americans with Disabilities Act (ADA), 27, 33–35
ANA*NET, 16
Anglo-American Cataloging Rules (AACR), 116
Anglo-American Cataloging Rules (AACR2R), *see* AACR2R (Anglo-American Cataloging Rules)
Annual reviews, management of, 80
AORN Journal, 19
Approval plans, 158–159
Architecture, LANs, 39–40
Archival materials, processing of, 193
Archival-quality, 250
Archival records:
arrangement of, 229–231
description of, 231–232
Archives, 219
Archives, Personal Papers and Manuscripts (APPM), 232
ARCnet, 38, 41
Armed Forces Medical Library, 306
Army Medical Library, 306
Arrangement(s):
archival records, 229–231
journals, 122
magazines, 122
of special collections, 229
Artifacts, 219
Assessment, collection, 167–170
Associate degree programs, 3
Association for College & Research Libraries, standards, 52–53
Association of Operating Room Nurses (AORN), 18
Association of Records Managers and Administrators (ARMA), 238

342

Index

Index

Index

Index

Index

Index

Index